PRAISE FOR IN THE GAPS

"This magnificent book transcends the divisiveness and rancor in current policies and attitudes toward homelessness in America. Humor, science, and wisdom are punctuated with unforgettable stories from the streets and shelters told by a brilliant and compassionate doctor who urges us to join a common journey toward understanding and ending the scourge of homelessness. This book will inflame your heart, stimulate your mind, and ultimately challenge us all to embrace our shared ideals of respect, altruism, and love for one another. Brace yourself for a breathtaking and radical journey."

—JIM O'CONNELL, MD, president, Boston Health Care for the Homeless, assistant professor, Harvard Medical School, and subject of *Rough Sleepers* by Tracy Kidder

"*In the Gaps* is a must-read...for everyone. From his firsthand perspective, Dr. Klausner weaves a story of the unhoused that humanizes those who perhaps bear the greatest brunt of society's ills, those that most of us choose not to see. His masterful analysis of root causes digs deep into racism, historical injustices, and enduring inequitable social structures. By moving beyond individual shortcomings, he forces us to see ourselves and the systems that we uphold in the solutions that can address homelessness and other big social problems. Though current generations did not cause these problems, we must act to solve them or be crushed by the cost of our inefficiencies. Brilliant!"

—LAURA GERALD, MD, MPH, president, Kate B. Reynolds Charitable Trust

"An important and illuminating book. With humanity and rigor, Dr. Brian Klausner takes readers on an engaging and at times heartrending journey to the front lines of chronic homelessness in America, sharing his experiences caring for some of the nation's most vulnerable patients and exploring the broader forces that are shaping this national crisis."

—**NOAM LEVEY, senior correspondent, KFF Health News**

"After wiping tears from my face numerous times, I had to process the stories and wisdom shared by Dr. Brian Klausner in this must-read book. Some takeaways: Our unsheltered community should not be judged or blamed, they should be helped. Yes, treating people is expensive, but it is more expensive if we take shortcuts. Finally, cities, counties, states, and the federal government need to work better together to address homelessness, prevent trauma, and ensure that more housing is built throughout our country. It's time we treat our unsheltered as human beings—because they are."

—**MARY-ANN BALDWIN, mayor of Raleigh, North Carolina**

"Whether you are a healthcare professional, a civic leader, or just someone who stares in disbelief at the plight of those living on the street, you need to read this book to truly understand where to start to fix the gaps in our humanity. Dr. Klausner has walked the walk—both literally on the streets and in boardrooms centered on the health and welfare of the unhoused. He gives us a guide for where we should be putting our resources and our hearts."

—**MATTHEW NATHAN, MD, former Surgeon General, United States Navy**

"Dr. Brian Klausner's compelling new book on providing healthcare to the unhoused will both open your eyes and break your heart. Through expert storytelling, Klausner illustrates how our healthcare system can both help and hurt this pervasive problem in our communities. From his two decades of working on the frontlines in Boston and Raleigh, Dr. Klausner humanizes the "statistics of suffering" and outlines compassionate solutions. Whether you are in the medical field or simply a concerned human, this book is essential reading for those of us wanting to understand the complexities of caring for the unhoused."

—**KATHY IZARD, author,** *The Hundred Story Home* **and** *Trust the Whisper*

"A compelling and immensely readable book about the plight of the forgotten from a doctor who has spent a lifetime knowing them."

—**SHANTANU NUNDY, MD, Chief Health Officer Accolade and author,** *Care After Covid*

"Dr. Brian Klausner's work is a testament to the profound beauty of human resilience. His ability to see beyond scars—both physical and emotional—and uncover the hidden strength within each individual is truly inspiring. In *In the Gaps*, he not only gives a voice to the overlooked but also celebrates the quiet, messy, and unyielding spirit that defines us all. His insights have deeply resonated with me as a fellow trauma survivor, reminding us that even in the darkest moments, there is a transformative power in our shared humanity."

—**JOSE PEREIRA, author,** *From Hero to Villain,* **five year hostage survivor, and member of the CITGO6**

IN THE GAPS

IN THE GAPS

BETTER UNDERSTANDING THE EXPENSIVE HUMAN SUFFERING OF CHRONIC HOMELESSNESS

BRIAN KLAUSNER, MD

SPIRITUS BOOKS

In the Gaps: Better Understanding the Expensive Human Suffering of Chronic Homelessness

Copyright © 2024 Brian Klausner, MD

All rights reserved

No part of this book may be reproduced in any form or by any electronic or mechanical means including information storage and retrieval systems, without permission in writing from the author. The only exception is by a reviewer, who may quote short excerpts in a published review.

Disclaimer: This book reflects the author's recollections and experiences. Some names have been changed or details limited or modified to protect privacy. Other events were omitted or compressed. Some dialogue was recreated. While every attempt has been made to verify the information in this book, the author does not assume any responsibility for errors, inaccuracies, or omissions. Nothing in this book is intended as medical advice.

Cover: *Homeless Jesus* sculpture used with permission from sculptor Timothy Schmalz

ISBN (hardcover): 978-1-957473-03-1
ISBN (paperback): 978-1-957473-00-0
ISBN (e-book): 978-1-957473-02-4

Library of Congress Control Number: 2024924289

Edited by: Jocelyn Carbonara
Cover design by: Adam Hay
Interior design by: Jenny Lisk

Published by Spiritus Books, Hillsborough, North Carolina

Love is strength.
Hate is weakness.
Be strong.

For Joanne Guarino, the strongest person I have ever known, and in gratitude for all the patients I've had the honor to learn from over the years.

CONTENTS

Foreword — xiii
Jim O'Connell, MD

Introduction — 1

PART I
BEAUTIFUL

1. Scars — 11

PART II
BLINDNESS

2. Mr. Spears — 17
3. Vocation — 31
4. The Costume — 41
5. The Red Pill — 45
6. Why? — 51
7. Invisible — 65
8. The Tapeworm — 71
9. Alone — 81
10. Scattered Safety Nets — 87
11. The Dichotomy — 91
12. Comfortably Broken — 95
13. Hotspotting — 101
14. Bloodletting and Dirty Hands — 111

PART III
THE TREES

15. Kids Camp — 119
16. Aha — 129
17. The Curmudgeon — 141
18. Neuroplasticity — 147

PART IV
THE FOREST

19. Reflexive Dehumanization	153
20. Social Hierarchy	161
21. Loneliness	169
22. Twenty-Seven Pounds of Chains	173
23. The Beam	177
24. The Four Rs	183
25. Listen	189
26. Feeding the Fire While Fighting the Flame	201
27. Disparities	205

PART V
SHARED ROOTS

28. Mental Health	213
29. Justice System	223
30. One Nation	233
31. Under God	243
32. Break Zone	253

PART VI
LOVE

| 33. In the End | 263 |
| 34. One Cognitive Thought | 269 |

Acknowledgments	273
The Medical "Geek-Out" Appendix	279
Notes	293
Bibliography	303
Thank You!	311
About the Author	315

FOREWORD

JIM O'CONNELL, MD

Brian Klausner and Joanne Guarino mesmerized the incoming Harvard medical and dental students in August of 2011. After receiving their white coats on the Longwood Quadrangle on the last day of orientation, the eager students crowded into the amphitheater at the Brigham and Women's Hospital for their traditional first encounter with patients. During the first half hour, they were awed by Dr. Bernard Kinane, a beloved pediatric pulmonologist, and a successful young accountant with a rare genetic disorder whom he had cared for since he was an infant three decades earlier. Dr. Klausner, who had worked with our Boston Health Care for the Homeless Program (BHCHP) for four memorable years and had flown in for this occasion from North Carolina, then introduced Joanne who had survived years on Boston's streets. Over the next 30 minutes, they gave a stunning master class on the mutual respect, endurance, and love that are at the heart of the doctor-patient relationship, the bedrock of the profession these aspiring doctors were about to enter.

After unspeakable trauma as a child and decades enduring harsh physical and sexual violence on the streets, Joanne met Dr. Klausner when he was a physician leading an integrated and multidisciplinary team caring for patients at our 104-bed Barbara McInnis House, a medical respite unit for homeless persons discharged from local hospitals but still too sick to withstand the rigors of surviving in shelters and on the streets. Joanne was startled by Dr. Klausner's gracious kindness, rapt listening, sincere compassion, and infectious humor. Together they embarked on a long journey, accompanying each other as Joanne faced the ravages of rheumatoid arthritis, pulmonary hypertension, and a bewildering cascade of medical, psychiatric, and substance use problems rendered immensely more challenging without the safety and security of stable housing. Joanne attributes her life to the devotion and care of Dr. Klausner, and proudly serves as a vibrant member of our program's Board of Directors as well as a local and national spokesperson for so many who have endured the social tragedy of homelessness.

Dr. Klausner inspired all of us during the years he worked with us in Boston. A brilliant and skilled physician and consummate team player, he worked not only at our respite program and our clinic in the city's 450-bed shelter located on Boston's Long Island, one of several islands in Boston Harbor, but also as the medical director who rapidly became the soul and inspiration of our busy Boston Medical Center clinic for homeless persons. His West Coast allegiance and suffocating love of the Los Angeles Lakers was obnoxious to us Bostonians. This even extended to a disdain of the quality of East Coast hot dogs. A self-professed connoisseur, Dr. Klausner endured a humbling epiphany when he stumbled across Speed Anderson's hot dog truck hidden in the meatpacking district just a short walk from our main clinic. Reluctantly conceding that Speed's was the best hot dog he had ever tasted, he soon became a Pied Piper leading our staff on regular lunch-hour pilgrimages to Speed's wagon, replete with laughter and incessant Boston/LA banter that brought much joy to all of us.

This remarkable book is the riveting *cri-de-coeur* of a skilled and compassionate doctor who cannot look away from the suffering, infections, chronic diseases, early death, and desperate loneliness he has witnessed firsthand for nearly two decades on the streets and in the shelters. Homelessness has become ubiquitous and seemingly intractable across the landscape of urban and rural America. A dearth of public and affordable housing is undoubtedly the root cause of this national tragedy. During the first meeting of the nascent Health Care for the Homeless Program of the Robert Wood Johnson Foundation in the fall of 1985, Cushing Dolbeare, the fiery founder of the National Low Income Housing Coalition, cautioned us to be wary of attributing homelessness to individual failures and found the metaphor of musical chairs most useful. When the music stops, those on crutches, distracted by inner voices, or facing other challenges are not able to compete equally and are left without a chair. While the cause of their homelessness is the lack of available chairs, left standing in this competition are those who struggle with institutional racism, income disparity, and structural failures. Weakness in sectors such as welfare, foster care, education, justice, labor, health, and public policy continue to pave the many roads that converge eventually in homelessness.

Dr. Klausner jolts the reader's understanding of homelessness through searing and unforgettable portraits of his resilient and courageous patients. A gifted and extraordinary storyteller, he scatters these narratives throughout the book to illustrate his arguments. Among the memorable are the gruff and paranoid Mr. Spears whose relationship with Dr. Klausner began with a curse and a sudden strike with his cane to move the doctor out of his way. Michele's descent into homelessness and addiction was precipitated by medical bills after a serious illness. Mike, who possessed nothing and lived in the parking lot behind Olive Garden, prayed each morning at 4 a.m. and found only beauty all around him as he was suffering from end-stage heart failure. Unforgettably, Dr. Klausner is called to see a 60-year-old woman with COVID wandering in a local park wearing 27 pounds of chains around her waist with multiple locks that served as a chastity belt to help cope with unspeakable sexual abuse and trauma in her past.

These stories punctuate Dr. Klausner's invaluable book and undermine any complacency about the societal disgrace of homelessness. He pleads for respectful political discourse and a collective willingness to face the burden of suffering on the streets and in the shelters of America. Without understanding, solutions are impossible. And as he so compellingly notes, the rush to solutions has been accompanied by growing numbers and profound—and expensive—suffering. Indeed, people living chronically without homes comprise a relatively small percentage of the United States population but account for nearly one-quarter of medical expenses in the United States, a number which he notes is close to one trillion dollars each year. He points to the irony of our health care system that professes allegiance to a Hippocratic Oath that directs us to treat all patients "to the best of our ability" yet excludes so many poor and vulnerable individuals. Poor understanding results in policies that punish those most in need, as exemplified by a justice system that further isolates people whose activities of daily living become "crimes of existence" when done in public.

Dr. Klausner laments the dehumanization that immunizes us from the suffering despite the call of virtually all great religions to care for the least among us. Reaching beyond the familiar moral, religious, and economic arguments to end homelessness, Dr. Klausner reviews the neurobiological literature that shatters our defensive postures and demonstrates the marked health benefits of caring rather than excluding.

Dr. Klausner's far-reaching and provocative journey concludes with a courageous appeal for love and compassion, precisely what he and Joanne Guarino exemplified for the Harvard students fifteen years ago. Mileposts throughout this must-read book foresee this appeal.

This magnificent book transcends the divisiveness and rancor in current policies and attitudes toward homelessness in America. Humor, science, and wisdom are punctuated with unforgettable stories from the streets and shelters told by a brilliant and compassionate doctor who urges us to join a common journey toward understanding and ending the scourge of homelessness. This book will inflame your heart, stimulate your mind, and ultimately challenge us all to embrace our shared ideals of respect, altruism, and love for one another. Brace yourself for a breathtaking and radical journey in the pages ahead.

Jim O'Connell, MD
President, Boston Health Care for the Homeless Program
Assistant Professor, Harvard Medical School
Department of Medicine, Massachusetts General Hospital
Subject of Tracy Kidder's *New York Times* bestseller *Rough Sleepers*

INTRODUCTION

Knowledge of mechanism is everything.

To be inhumane is one thing. To be inefficient is another. With our approach to chronic homelessness in America, we are both.

This isn't a political statement or a social commentary. It's more of a diagnosis—one that I stubbornly missed for years.

If we're truthful, most of us can admit to a discrepancy between our daily actions and the ideals we aspire to that are preached in our congregations, schools, living rooms, and mission statements. Within these hypocritical gaps between our words and our actions, you'll find the expensive and preventable suffering of a misunderstood population as well as the dysfunctional hemorrhaging of taxpayer money.

In my years as a doctor working with patients experiencing homelessness, I have worked in these gaps—and been honored to get to know incredible people with incredible strength as they battle impossible odds to maintain their health ... or simply survive. I have been inspired by their stubborn resilience and daily determination for a better life. And I have watched too many of them lose their lonely battles. Most didn't suffer and die cheaply. Almost all died misunderstood—both by others and by themselves.

These patients I've known were brothers and sisters, mothers and fathers, wives and husbands. They were cousins, coworkers, neighbors, former childhood best friends, teammates, and first loves. They were all sons or daughters who at one time shared, at least to some extent, in the hopes and dreams of youth that never materialized as their worlds grew progressively darker around them.

Their histories often included trauma, shattered dreams, broken relationships, illness, and loneliness. Most of the chronically homeless patients I've cared for have battled complex pathologies with clinical manifestations that have decreased their years on Earth while isolating them from families and friends who either wouldn't, or more likely couldn't, help them. These pathologies were often rooted in early and even cross-generational trauma that firmly and tragically established their life trajectories toward this suffering.

Their strength fighting against these trajectories is inspiring. Our costly failures to efficiently assist them are haunting.

As patients, those suffering from homelessness have overwhelmed an American healthcare system that swore a Hippocratic Oath to treat all patients to the "best of our ability" yet has never tried very hard to provide its actual best specifically for *them*. Instead of being helped, they're often blamed and judged for their pathologies by medical systems more focused on maximizing efficiency and profitability in healthier and wealthier populations.

As a physician who trained in this American healthcare system and accidentally stumbled into a career in homeless medicine, my journey has been one of constant aha moments. I've often discovered key lessons only through the clarity of hindsight after it was too late to help the patients who taught me. Perhaps these were better characterized as *Sixth Sense* moments, wherein I became suddenly aware of realities that were in front of me the entire time.

Working in these gaps, often blindly, I have misunderstood. I have blamed. I have committed medicine's cardinal sin of chasing symptoms instead of addressing root causes. But I have also learned —slowly. I have witnessed patients experience incredible hard-won success, and I have celebrated with them as they moved out of the chaos and trauma of chronic homelessness. Admittedly, in my career, I have found that failures tend to be more haunting than successes are inspiring, but both provide motivation to continue to do better.

As we work to address the growing issues around homelessness in our society, the expensive gaps between our words and actions should not be ignored or defensively dismissed. Instead, they should be studied, dissected, and better understood. Knowledge is the antidote to the dysfunction of ignorance. If we can better understand, down to the neurobiological level, the human behaviors that underlie homelessness on one hand, and those that drive the discrepancies between our societal words and actions on the other, we can more effectively address root causes. If we look carefully and listen honestly, we can identify genuine opportunities—bipartisan opportunities—to create a more humane and efficient society. When this becomes our goal and focus, *opportunity* quickly becomes synonymous with *obligation*.

I recently visited my hometown of Los Angeles for the first time in years. Driving down the streets leading to my old high school, I saw seemingly endless rows of tents, cardboard boxes, and lived-in cars that served as "homes" for tens of thousands of city residents. The homeless crisis continues to grow across our nation as numbers reach record highs.[1] Over the decades, as rent has increased and affordable housing options have shrunk, homelessness in our nation has progressively worsened. This issue now paralyzes many communities, especially in larger cities like Los Angeles—becoming a major concern for residents and a central focus in local elections.

The main current driver of homelessness is not mental illness or addiction; it is simply supply and demand of affordable housing. The cost of housing has reached a level where many people simply cannot afford it.

Residents in larger cities are demanding solutions, but they often avoid options that could negatively impact them personally—such as zoning laws or affordable housing projects in their own neighborhoods that might affect their home prices. Yet social policies and increased affordable housing are crucial if we are to work toward the United States Interagency Council on Homelessness's goal of making homelessness "rare, brief, and one time."[2] We must face this rising prevalence of short-term homelessness in the context of a lack of affordable housing. However, as we do so, we must simultaneously improve strategies to assist those suffering from *chronic* homelessness, defined as "people who have experienced homelessness for at least a year—or repeatedly—while struggling with a disabling condition such as a serious mental illness, substance use disorder, or physical disability."[3] These are individuals who are not able to escape from temporary homelessness, instead getting stuck in its expensive—and often fatal—chronic state. The severity of their underlying pathologies, and the inefficiencies of our response, consume our increasingly limited resources.

There is an urgency to become more efficient and targeted in how we manage the medical and mental health conditions in individuals who suffer from chronic homelessness. This will take a village, truly, and require a much greater level of collaboration between the historically siloed sectors of social services, healthcare, and local governments. We'll need more data and analytics to shine a bright, persistent light on the financial cost of our inefficiencies, making them impossible to keep ignoring, while better guiding our policies and associated legislation.

In medicine, specifically, we'll need to practice more patience as we strive for smarter, more evidenced-based, and much more innovative solutions in our patient care. While historically our performance in managing homeless populations doesn't provide much reason for optimism, recent pressures and payment-reform models in healthcare provide motivation and potential glimpses of hope for improvement. With healthcare costs in America now well over $4 trillion a year and consuming nearly 20 percent of our GDP,[4] we simply can no longer afford to mismanage high-risk patient populations.

It is not about politics. It's not conservative or liberal. It's not even, really, about humanity—or at least it doesn't need to be. It can be simply about creating greater efficiency, which makes it, surprisingly in today's world, uniquely bipartisan … if we are smart. And there is an urgent need for us to be smart and stop hemorrhaging taxpayer money on avoidable human suffering.

This is not a book necessarily about solving homelessness. It is a book, hopefully, about better understanding it.

I tried not to make it a memoir, but I do start the book by sharing my personal journey of how I stumbled into a career caring for patients experiencing homelessness, fighting through my own stereotypes and misconceptions to better understand how to help them.

I then move on to discuss how our medical teams evolved to better understand the root causes of chronic homelessness—at an individual level, but more importantly at our collective societal level. The book explores how our pathologies as an American healthcare system have resulted in our failures to efficiently address the expensive suffering of chronic homelessness. It then goes on to demonstrate how these pathologies are shared by other sectors of our society that impact homelessness. The science behind these societal pathologies is fascinating—and important, if we are to learn to do better.

Knowledge of mechanism is everything. If we hope to efficiently address the growing issues around homelessness in our nation—and its associated costs—we'll need a better understanding of its underlying pathologies. Even in our increasingly partisan and polarized society, there is the potential for us to be much more humane and efficient by striving to better live up to the common ideals and beliefs that most of us share.

That is what this book is about. (We will see how I did …)

Of note, when I started writing this book years ago, I was initially focused on the medical field as a target audience. However, as I increasingly realized that our inefficiencies in medicine caring for those experiencing chronic homelessness are symptoms of larger human tendencies and predispositions, I shifted the focus to a more general population. But I could not resist the temptation to "geek out" occasionally throughout the book by getting into more detail on topics that may interest a medical audience. I have marked these instances and placed them in an appendix section for those who are interested in delving deeper into these topics.

Most of the patients I'll discuss in this book are, sadly, deceased. This is almost an inevitability when working with a chronically homeless population where the life expectancy still hovers around 50. I try hard to remember their names, their stories, and the lessons each taught me, afraid that if I don't, the memories of these incredible people will be forgotten entirely from this world. As street artist Banksy once wrote: "They say you die twice. Once when you stop breathing and the second, a bit later on, when somebody mentions your name for the last time." I could not prevent their first death, so perhaps as a coping mechanism, I work to prevent their second. There is something to that—especially if it brings progress in how we care for future patients.

To continue protecting the confidentiality of my patients, however, I won't use their actual names and may change some of the details of their history; but hopefully their stories of suffering and strength will honor their memories and provide insights into how we can do better in the future. Their stories are powerful enough that no fabrication or embellishment is needed. In fact, I've been intentional in leaving out some of their life details and trauma, as I don't believe they ever intended those stories to be shared, even anonymously.

The exception to this anonymity is Joanne Guarino, who has agreed to let me share her story. After experiencing homelessness on and off for 30 years, she has become a speaker, mentor, and supporter of solutions through her work with multiple advocacy groups. This is why I have dedicated this book to her—because of her strength, love, brilliance, and persistent thick-south-Boston-don't-pronounce-my-hard-Rs-accented determination to pull people out of the expensive hypocritical gaps of our society as she works tirelessly to erase those gaps altogether.

PART I
BEAUTIFUL

1

SCARS

There is nothing more beautiful than human resilience.

He walked into my clinic smiling, in good spirits and well-dressed with sunglasses. He'd flown in late the night before, but he reported that he still was able to get a great night's sleep at the hotel up the street. After having coffee at the trendy, free-wi-fi, indie-music-playing coffee shop across the street, he was ready for our visit.

As we walked back to the corner clinic—I always made sure to reserve our only exam room with a window—we made small talk about the nice weather that day in Raleigh and his pleasant experience at RDU airport, which, he marveled, contrasted greatly with his much larger airport back home. After taking his vitals, I asked about his past medical history, his family's medical history, and previous medications he'd taken. I had learned by that time to let the stories of recent captivity come up naturally as the conversation evolved—and they always did.

"I was completely healthy before *it* happened ..." The door had opened.

The conversation quickly went into the details of his years in captivity overseas, which had just ended two months prior, providing a dark contrast to the pleasant small talk that had started our interaction. He began with the day of his capture. He had been in the country visiting his family and took a simple trip to a local gas station. He described his initial surprise when he was grabbed by a group of masked men, followed by the horror of realizing what was happening. And then ... a constant nightmare that lasted over four years but felt like an eternity.

The details of his stories in captivity were just as horrific as what you would see in the movies—or worse.

It was the *persistence* of his trauma and pain that was so striking. The horror wasn't just in few-minute segments augmented by music and dramatic camera shots. It was constant and brutal. Relentless.

Our team at WakeMed made the decision to clinically partner with Hostage US back in 2019. Each year, an estimated 200 Americans on average are taken hostage or wrongly detained overseas—often quietly, as any publicity or attention runs the risk of making conditions worse for them. Hostage US is an amazing nonprofit that assists American captives who were held overseas as they attempt to reassimilate back into their lives after being released or rescued. We are one of two hospital partners affiliated with the program. Clients typically come in for a three-day extensive medical and behavioral health evaluation and treatment.

I believed we could contribute to Hostage US given our experience with trauma-informed clinical models. However, I was cautious entering into our partnership, knowing that we were still novices, and the extent of the trauma their clients endured would be extreme and prolonged.

That day in clinic, he struggled at different points when talking about the physical torture he'd suffered and the injuries his captors had caused. Twice, he broke down in tears.

We arrange for this first clinic visit to be 90 minutes to allow patients plenty of time to share their stories. Then, after a 15 to 20 minute coffee break or walk outside for the patient, their initial visit with me is followed by a 90-minute appointment with our trauma therapist.

As I started on the physical exam, the findings gave testimony to his suffering—suddenly bringing a stark reality to these stories of torture and captivity in lands far away from our downtown Raleigh clinic. Scars from where he was routinely electrocuted, "almost for fun" by one particularly psychopathic-ish guard. Scars from where he'd been beaten and whipped. He couldn't fully raise his shoulders due to being hung by chains during many of those beatings. An MRI the next day would reveal bilateral rotator cuff tears. (This type of injury is something we would repeatedly see in our Hostage US patients.) His fingers were deformed from multiple fractures.

Yet he—like all the other patients I've served through the program—didn't identify the actual physical trauma as the worst part of his experience or as what continued to haunt him. It was not *what* was done to him, but *how* it was done that caused the most pain —and continued to paralyze him. How could other humans look him in the eye and repeatedly do these things to him—treating him with such blatant disregard? It was the painful memories of being persistently treated like he was less than human that tortured him the most, not the physical injuries. His PTSD flashbacks and the nightmares that kept him up at night revolved around the dehumanizing glances and stares, not the beatings.

I have found it difficult to put myself "in the shoes" of our Hostage US clients. I can try to imagine a few minutes, or maybe even hours, of torture or trauma. But to extend that suffering as it drags on for weeks, months, or years on end? Violent. Alone. Constant. That existence feels impossible to comprehend.

How did he survive? I asked myself. *How?*

His resilience was definitely inspirational; it was also very familiar from my work caring for patients experiencing chronic homelessness.

As humans, we love conflict, drama, and fiction along with all of their heroes. We are often as drawn to the characters' inspirational determination to fight as we are to their ultimate success. Yet strangely, we're often blind to the resilience of people we encounter in our daily lives, which frequently dwarfs anything found in meticulously crafted fiction.

Perhaps this is because, in reality, resilience can be so subtle and quiet, not accentuated by dramatic music or narrated with perfectly written scripts. It is sloppy and improvised.

Perhaps it is because the greatest displays of human strength and beauty are often buried under the scars of time, hidden and disguised. Frequently, these scars are so deep and ugly that we reflexively look away, misinterpreting them as the ultimate reality while ignoring the beauty they're obscuring.

There is nothing more beautiful than human resilience. It is a shame when we are blind to it.

PART II
BLINDNESS

2

MR. SPEARS

Early in my career, I loved practicing medicine in the hospital setting. Perhaps I was drawn to the familiarity from years as a medical student and then as a resident, where hospitals served as our main teaching environment. Even in the exhaustion and stress of my training, I appreciated the important work of those battling tirelessly inside the hospital's walls. The illnesses treated and lives saved. The daily application of scientific knowledge and advancements to benefit our patients. The amazing technology supporting their care. Our work was incredibly hard, and for the most part, we did it well. People came to the hospital sick and, typically, left healthier. What happened inside the hospital's walls was often life-changing for many, and even life-saving for some.

My first job out of residency was with Boston Health Care for the Homeless Program (BHCHP). For a few weeks each year, physicians in the program would leave their outpatient clinics to manage inpatient teaching services at local hospitals. This allowed us to stay current with hospital medicine in academic environments while keeping an eye on BHCHP patients who were sick in the hospital. I was almost a year into my position with BHCHP when I did my first rotation as an attending physician—overseeing a team of medical residents and students.

The first few days of my rotation went well, with challenging cases presenting great teaching opportunities. I loved getting back to my familiar clinical comfort zone: inpatient academic medicine, where everything was more controlled and supported by large clinical teams.

For much of my preceding first year at BHCHP, I had felt relatively lost. The vast majority of my training in medical school and my residency was in hospital settings. This was the norm at the time—and for most training programs, it still is today. This setup benefits physicians who choose careers in inpatient medicine, but not necessarily the young doctors who want to practice outpatient medicine. Pathologies and diseases develop and progress in the community—outside of the controlled environment of the hospital, during the 99.9 percent of the time they are not in our medical settings but rather living their day-to-day lives. I'd learned to algorithmically manage diseases in my residency and in my board exams, but the application of these algorithms became much more confusing when filtered through the real-world chaos of homelessness.

When evidence-based medical algorithms get disrupted by the uncertain realities of patients' social situations, clinicians must improvise and compromise. These are not skills that are taught in books or classes. They are ones that veteran providers at BHCHP developed over the years through experience.

I quickly came to realize that, during the eight years of medical training preceding my first job at BHCHP, I'd learned the science of medicine without ever really learning its *art*—how to apply the science to each individual's unique needs and circumstances to maximize their outcomes. The *science* of medicine revolves around us as providers. The *art* of medicine revolves around the patient. While knowing the science is a necessary prerequisite to successfully applying the art, it's only one part. After confidently strolling out of my chief residency the year prior, I was quickly humbled by needing to come to grips with this.

Over the next four years at BCHCP, the nurses, providers, and other staff members around me taught me this art of medicine. Fortunately, they were experts. In fact, the humbling of arrogant young doctors was kind of a rite of passage with BHCHP. Luckily, the supportive environment there made it easy to learn while not shattering egos.

Being back in the hospital, however, it felt like I did not need to worry about any of this. I could get back to the algorithms I'd mastered and taught in my chief residency year. There was control and comfort inside the hospital walls. I loved it.

I'd gotten extremely lucky with my teaching team for this particular rotation. Mark, an experienced senior resident, led the team of two energetic interns and a couple of incredible students.

One morning, a week into my attending rotation, on my way to meet my team for rounds, I quickly stopped by the room of a patient who was set for an early discharge. I intended to say goodbye and answer any questions. She and her husband had been visiting from Pennsylvania to spend a weekend with their daughter in college. As they were driving to a football game on a Saturday morning, she developed crushing chest pain. Fortunately, her husband kept on driving past the stadium and right to the hospital. Within 90 minutes from the onset of her symptoms, still with a temporary tattoo of her daughter's school on her cheek, she had a stent successfully placed in one of her coronary arteries that had been completely clogged by a ruptured plaque. Now a few days later, she felt great, her symptoms had resolved, and there was no apparent damage done to her heart. She and her husband were relieved and thankful. They went on and on about how lucky they felt to be in Boston, with all our great medical institutions, when this happened to her. They lived "in the sticks." They felt it was providence.

As we talked in her room, celebrating her success and the perceived efficiency of her care, I looked out of her window onto Albany Street, and my eye caught our new BHCHP headquarters.

Earlier that year, following a successful capital campaign, BHCHP had completed renovations on the old Boston city morgue, transforming it into our new headquarters. The building was beautiful. On the first floor was Jean Yawkey Place, named after a legendary longtime Boston Red Sox owner and local philanthropist. The state-of-the-art medical, mental-health, and dental clinics, as well as an outpatient pharmacy, were truly all game changers in eliminating many of the access barriers BHCHP had historically faced with providing care. On the second and third floors were the 104 beds for our respite care center. These were essentially "step-down beds" for patients who were too sick to be in the streets or shelters, but not sick enough to necessitate remaining in the hospital. It was an incredible model that would save a lot of money ... and lives.

The building had just opened a few months before, bringing immense excitement and pride to our organization while expanding our clinical capabilities. That morning, the autumn foliage was in full bloom—which, in South Boston, meant that the occasional tree on Massachusetts Avenue tried hard to add color and a sense of nature to an otherwise very urban landscape.

On the streets, I could already see some familiar faces in their daily routines. Ms. Johnson was struggling with the incredible numbers of bags she somehow managed to carry despite the severe arthritis in her back. Kevin was already on his usual street corner, panhandling. He was never too successful, as his loud and constant external responses to the several different voices he heard in his head scared off most potential donors. And there was Joyce, hanging out on our side-door stoop, where she would often wait until our clinic opened to patients at 8 a.m. I felt glad to see her, since she had left our respite facility a week before, despite our pleas to stay as she was still recovering from pneumonia.

I said my goodbyes to my patient and her husband and navigated a series of hallways to meet the residents and students so we could start morning rounds. The hospital seemed to be humming with its normal clinical efficiency. Nurses navigating their carts around the halls, delivering medications, addressing alarm monitors, and obtaining vitals. Medical students and residents preparing notes and writing orders. Patients being educated about their care plans for the day. Everybody knowing their roles and positions in this well-orchestrated (and well-reimbursed) clinical dance. It was very impressive and always brought a definite sense of pride for all of us who participated.

As I approached my team of residents and students at the end of the long hallway, a sound suddenly broke through the efficient hum.

"Get the fuck away from me!"

Loud and clear, the command bellowed out of the room my team was standing in front of. It seemed particularly harsh this morning at 6:30 a.m., especially just after the special kumbaya-ish stare-out-the-window-at-the-autumn-foliage moment I'd shared with my patient. A few seconds later, a frightened medical student scurried out of the room, his eyes wide and his face blushing, as everybody had stopped their clinical dance to see what had happened.

It was only six words, but I recognized the voice right away—even before the complementary longer rant, with more choice words, that followed.

The voice was gruff, hoarse, and with a thick Boston accent. Booming and intimidating, it was familiar to me. The previous winter, this voice was the first thing I'd heard right *after* being surprised with a smack from the cane of its owner.

The senior resident, Mark, came out of the room soon after looking exhausted, which, even after hearing the outburst coming from the room, still surprised me. Mark was one of the best residents I'd ever worked with. He'd already received numerous intern and resident awards by the time we were on rotation together. Mark was dynamic, kind, personable, and extremely intelligent—which made his genuine humility even more impressive. He possessed an amazing ability to connect with patients, making them feel comfortable and then leveraging these connections into excellent patient care and outcomes.

On our daily morning rounds, we would discuss patient care plans and teach our interns and students about the diseases we were managing. I'd quickly perfected the art of looking like I was agreeing with Mark rather than learning from him as he taught the team (and me) something new or discussed some study I'd never read. The pace of medical knowledge evolves so quickly that it becomes almost impossible to keep up with unless you're constantly in it. As attending physicians, it's not uncommon to learn more from students and residents than we could ever teach them—but we just can't ever admit it.

This morning, Mark looked absolutely exhausted.

It also was not unusual for residents to be exhausted after a night on call; in fact, this was the norm. Medical residencies, at that time in 2008, were built around the overnight rotating call system. Every three or four nights, a resident's team would stay at the hospital—admitting new, sick patients and covering the patients of the other teams who weren't on call for that night. This routinely led to incredibly busy and almost always sleepless nights. But it brought a great opportunity to learn in a fast-paced baptism-by-fire environment. Still, the ensuing exhaustion could be brutal—so much so that increasing regulations and rules were enacted to provide a better balance and improve safety.

One of the most incredible aspects of being a young attending was no longer having to stay for overnight calls. Attending physicians could go home at night, taking occasional phone calls from residents to discuss any issues with new or existing patients. And we could do this guilt-free, as we'd put in our time as residents.

Part of the process involved exaggerating our experiences to fatigued residents in order to make them seem comparatively harder than theirs—just in case they were thinking about complaining. This allowed us, like I did that morning, to stroll in well-rested and showered while the overnight team was still essentially in the long, continuous workday we'd left them in the evening before. As a new attending physician, I appreciated this rite of passage as I recovered from the recent trauma of my own medical training.

Mark, before this, had never seemed flustered or tired. In fact, his routine typically involved taking time for a morning shower after his overnight call—in the cramped small resident bathroom—and arriving dressed in a shirt and tie instead of his overnight scrubs.

Nobody else did that, but Mark did, consistent with his overall professional, likable, and unflappable image.

That morning, however, things were different. He looked physically drained and thrown off his game (although still showered). Clearly he'd had a rough night. I wish my first instinct had been one of support and compassion, but truly it was more fascination over the details of what had happened.

"Mr. Spears?" I asked Mark as I approached, already knowing the answer.

"Yup," he replied, exhausted but seemingly relieved that I was familiar with the patient—removing him from the impossible task of describing just how challenging this patient was. I already knew.

Mr. Spears was much less intimidating physically than his booming, typically profanity-dishing voice. A small man—perhaps 5'5"—he had a thick beard and an emphysema-ish, barrel-chested, thin body. He slept outside, never staying in shelters. This resulted in his characteristically disheveled look and very poor hygiene, since he never really had the opportunity to take a shower. The impact of years of chronic homelessness had made him appear much older than his actual age.

Mr. Spears was a survivor, already outliving the life expectancy of chronically homeless individuals in America as he approached his late 50s. He was also paranoid, delusional, and constantly angry. All of this resulted in him being completely alone on the streets—no family, friend groups, or support. He could go days without anybody really even talking to him or saying his name, reinforcing a social isolation that only worsened his underlying mental health issues.

Mr. Spears would come in occasionally and reluctantly to our outpatient clinic for socks or clothes. Occasionally he would bring a medical complaint.

The previous winter, I'd seen him at our old outpatient clinic located on the first floor of the Boston Medical Center. He presented that day with a mild case of trench foot. This was a common, and deadly, condition seen during the trench warfare of WWI—when soldiers would sit for days in wet socks. Trench foot can become dangerous in a hurry due to associated infections, so early and adequate treatment is necessary. During the war, it killed thousands of soldiers. Today, trench foot really only affects unhoused populations living in chronically wet conditions without the ability to routinely change their socks.

That day in clinic, Mr. Spears had made it clear he wasn't coming into our respite care center for treatment—a common approach we used to get people off the streets, and out of their socks, as we provided skin treatments and prevented infection. His case was fortunately early and mild, so it was a relatively straightforward interaction. We provided several pairs of dry socks, some ointment, and clinical recommendations. We asked/begged him to follow up, so we could monitor his condition in the clinic. I sensed no tension or conflict. The entire visit seemed very straightforward. Which is why I was so surprised when he unexpectedly smacked me with his cane while exiting the room.

"Move!" he yelled, *after* he hit me. Common decency—and cane-smacking etiquette—would seem to dictate that one shouts the warning *before* applying the smack, if only by just a few seconds, and then only proceeds to strike if the verbal warning doesn't get the desired response. But not Mr. Spears; he reversed it. I'm still unsure why he did it, as my chair was as close to the desk as possible, giving him ample room to leave the clinic. It was only a mild wap—more of a reflex than an intentional act of violence. But whatever it was, something had triggered him. He loudly left the clinic, dishing out some F-bombs along the way, but at least grabbing the cream I'd given him as he headed back to the cold, snowy Boston winter that would inevitably worsen his trench foot, leading to a hospital admission a few weeks later.

"So, what's going on with Mr. Spears?" I asked Mark.

It was Mark's turn to be reflexive and emotional. His answer was a stark contrast to his normal, clinically brilliant, and award-winning humanistic baseline: "He's an ass."

Again, I wish I could say that my initial response was more appropriate—showing sympathy mixed with a firm reprimand—but instead all I felt was fascination. Mr. Spears had *broken* Mark the Resident.

After pausing for a few seconds and seeing the opportunity in front of me, I quickly composed myself. Tough cases always present the best teaching opportunities. When cases follow their expected course, they're quickly forgotten. It's the challenging cases that we learn from and remember. Mr. Spears had presented a teaching opportunity for everybody: Mark, the first-year interns, and the impressionable third-year medical students who'd just heard their role-model senior resident label the sick patient under his care as "an ass."

"Tell me what happened," I simply replied.

A prepared third-year student stepped in to share details in her well-rehearsed presentation ...

Mr. Spears was brought in late the previous night to our ER via ambulance. He'd just purchased groceries at a local store prior to feeling faint, becoming short of breath, and collapsing. The staff called 911. Upon arrival, the EMT team found Mr. Spears just outside of the store, trying hard to walk away but still very short of breath and weak—so weak he didn't resist being taken to the hospital. In the ER, he was found to have atrial fibrillation with "rapid ventricular response." This is a relatively common, and easily treated, arrhythmia that results in a rapid heart rate. In his case, it was fast enough and long enough that it was starting to stress his heart. His blood work was positive for cardiac enzymes, demonstrating that some of his heart cells were starting to die, unable to keep up with the demand of this elevated heart rate. While his enzymes, thankfully, were only mildly elevated, they still signaled an urgency to slow down his heart. An urgency that Mr. Spears wasn't really feeling.

Instead, all night, various attempts by residents, nurses, and consulting cardiologists to slow down his racing heart conflicted with Mr. Spears's immediate personal focus: protecting the bag of meat he'd purchased before collapsing at the grocery store. The EMT notes from the field reported he'd insisted on clutching the bag of meat during his entire transport, being "verbally abusive and aggressive" to anybody who tried to take it from him. Staff throughout the night worked to convince Mr. Spears to comply with medical care, initially with great patience, and then increasingly with great frustration.

Offers to place the meat in a refrigerator for safe keeping were met with profanities and vague threats, as were attempts to turn off alarms, administer medications, or change IV bags. Nothing was easy.

Psychiatry was later consulted and determined he was competent to make these decisions, no matter how poorly he chose. He fell into a frequently encountered gap of "competent enough to be determined competent legally, yet not competent enough to actually *be* competent," to possess the cognitive abilities to truly make good decisions about his health.

After the cane accident in the clinic a few months earlier, I had discussed Mr. Spears's case with one of our longtime psychiatrists. She'd only had brief, sporadic, and therefore ineffective interactions with him throughout the years. He'd had no interest in talking with her or working with anybody. His delusions, paranoia, and reflexive social agitation presented insurmountable barriers for even the best mental health providers.

Still, she learned that he had one of the worst histories of abuse as a child she'd ever seen—and she'd seen a lot. After his mother died early, he was raised by a father who suffered from addiction and subjected him to numerous forms of severe abuse, a pattern reinforced by random family members who resided with them over the years. His childhood was one of social isolation and fear, especially of an uncle who abused him in ways that were horrific and almost incomprehensible to anyone—except for him. He had no choice but to experience it.

Alone.

Instead of a childhood of love, support, and nurturing from caring adults, he was simply provided trauma and suffering. He was forced to try to grow up in that environment.

As the student presented his case, I quickly informed the team of this history of abuse to help round out his social history. Like education levels and past work experiences, this sort of history could help contextualize who a patient was, while sometimes providing clues to their clinical issues. At the time, I grasped this only as a contributing factor, while missing it as a physiological root cause.

After hearing the medical student's summary and witnessing Mark's uncharacteristically unprofessional behavior, I saw my opening. I excitedly ran to jump on my moral high horse.

I went on to explain to Mark, in front of the team, that while I recognized this was an extremely frustrating case, we must abide by an absolute rule: "We can never blame the patients for the pathologies they suffer from."

I continued to preach for a few more minutes, ending with, "Our job is to treat pathologies, even when they are difficult—*especially* when they are difficult—not whine about them." In hindsight, I probably went over the top, but I felt somewhat obligated to lay on the guilt a little; after all, you can't just call a patient "an ass."

Mark, through his fatigue and frustration, seemed to absorb the message with grace. Our rounds continued.

After we saw our other patients, I returned with our medical students to Mr. Spears, hoping that he'd had enough time to cool off. I made sure we kept our distance, even though the cane was not near his bed. I'd already learned Mr. Spears could move quickly when he wanted to.

"If we can't lower your heart rate, your heart will be in danger," I started after failed attempts at small talk. As I spoke, his monitor continued to beep loudly, demonstrating a rate of around 130 beats per minute. However, reasoning with him was truly an exercise in futility. He wasn't listening; he was reacting. I couldn't calm him down enough to agree to our rational and relatively algorithmic plan, which would include taking routinely used medications to slow his heart rate.

I kept talking about his heart rate and cardiac enzymes. He kept yelling about the bag of meat in the corner of the room. He still wouldn't let anybody touch it or refrigerate it for him. It was already growing rancid, further disrupting and stinking up the normally efficient morning hospital routine. As he became more entrenched in his stubbornness, I reflexively escalated my messaging around urgency and dangers.

More than an hour later, we were further apart than when we had started. I felt myself reacting instead of thinking. Occasionally, my team would pop in to sign orders, check vitals, and watch my "progress."

We kept working with him throughout the morning until suddenly he got up, tore off his beeping monitors, grabbed his cane and bag of rancid meat, and started to leave—loudly. He paused only briefly to give two silent middle fingers to the requests that he sign the "against medical advice" forms.

Mark was at the nurses' station, writing notes and orders, as Mr. Spears busted out of his room. Mark looked up from his position, which was close enough to have heard my final desperate attempts with Mr. Spears—and, likely, the loud "thud" of me falling off my high horse.

While other staff members exchanged nervous smiles and subtle eye-rolling in response to the awkwardness of the situation as Mr. Spears left the floor, Mark's face only demonstrated genuine concern. True to form, he showed no evidence of smugness. It had to be there somewhere, but if it was, he didn't show it. He had enough insight to appreciate what was playing out in front of him—that we were getting our asses kicked by a pathology we didn't know how to address.

As a physician, it is haunting to watch severe pathology walk out the door untreated. For the most part, when discharged into the community, it will inevitably return—victorious either in death or in a much more advanced, severe, and expensive state.

The latter was the case with Mr. Spears, who was admitted a few days later into our ICU after collapsing again in the community.

Mr. Spears would die a few years later on the streets, beating the average age of death for those who suffer from chronic homelessness by almost 10 years.[1] This was a truly remarkable feat and a tribute to his stubborn determination, considering the number and severity of pathologies life threw his way—which violently and expensively defied our ability and efforts to help him.

The rest of the inpatient rotation got back on track after that one eventful morning with Mr. Spears. Many of our cases were fascinating, with good outcomes. Of all the patients we treated during our time together, however, I think (and hope) the team learned the most from Mr. Spears. Often the greatest teaching moments in medicine come in the form of defeat. We just have to be humble enough, as we get knocked off our self-absorbed high horses, to recognize them.

3

VOCATION

Practicing medicine for those experiencing homelessness was not a lifelong dream of mine. Becoming a doctor was not even on my radar when starting college. Entering my first year at Notre Dame in 1993, I had no idea what I wanted to do with my life. I felt relatively directionless as I attempted to select a major. I ultimately decided on mechanical engineering, following my parents' advice that if I did, at least I'd "learn how to think."

They were right. I "learned to think" that I didn't want to go into engineering. There were times, especially in my first-year Engineering Calculus class, when I was convinced people were just messing with me—that it was all some big practical joke or a hidden-camera TV show. There was no way anybody could actually understand what was being taught.

However, for as much as I disliked my engineering classes, I found that I enjoyed both my entry-level chemistry and biology classes. By the end of my first year, I had selected a major in biology.

My sophomore year, I took the dreaded but required organic chemistry. This served as a weed-out course for the many science and pre-med students at Notre Dame interested in medical school.

Perhaps not having that particular goal at that particular time allowed me to be more relaxed than my peers. I was surprised to find that the class most students feared, I enjoyed—in kind of a nerdy, actually-had-fun-studying type of way. At the time, doing well in organic chemistry suggested one should at least consider going into medicine. More than 25 years later, I'm not exactly sure why that was, as I have never really used organic chemistry since that time. Whatever it was, I fell for it. My interest and relative success in organic chemistry made me, for the first time, consider becoming a physician.

Fortunately, I had a role model from whom I could seek guidance.

My grandfather was an old-school, Normal Rockwell-ish family physician—black bag and all. He received his degree from Northwestern Medical School in the early 1930s, marrying my grandmother during his last year of training. After graduation and residency, they returned to Los Angeles, where they both had grown up and attended UCLA for college. He set up a private practice toward the end of the Great Depression. To make ends meet financially, he also worked as a "police surgeon" with the Los Angeles Receiving Hospital—treating trauma victims both in the hospital and on the streets while rounding with the police units.

His young career was disrupted when he was called to serve in WWII and left his wife and four children to provide medical care to troops in the South Pacific. My father wasn't quite one year old when his father left. He was three by the time he came back home. My grandfather returned to his clinic in Los Angeles after the war, picking up where he'd left off. He would happily continue his traditional office-based practice for decades.

In their mid-80s, he and my grandmother moved to a retirement home in Santa Barbara, tucked between the Pacific coast and the Santa Ynez Mountains. When my grandmother passed away a few months after their 60th wedding anniversary, my grandfather's four kids and 19 grandchildren would make frequent trips to visit him. I tried to travel to see him a few times per year—sometimes with my older siblings, sometimes by myself.

Our typical visits would involve sitting in the living room of his apartment with his windows open, allowing the ocean breeze to blow in as we talked for hours. Outside of his room, a fountain in the courtyard koi pond added to the calming ambiance. Those visits became nostalgic to me, with no phones, no texting, no distraction—nothing but conversation with a man who had led an incredible life and was eager to pass on the knowledge and insights to his family before his time came to an end.

He, like so many of his generation, was an incredible storyteller. He would effortlessly transition from one story to another, often focusing on his incredible career in a medical field that he loved.

He was the quintessential *general* practitioner—an ER, OB/GYN, pediatrician, geriatrician, cardiologist, GI, etc., doctor all rolled into one—and he stubbornly remained that way his entire career. Following WWII, specialization in medicine proliferated. Expanding medical knowledge, new technologies, and new treatments pushed more doctors away from the generalist role and into specific medical specialties, and then subspecialties. The growth and federal support of hospitals—increasingly seen as essential, lifesaving centers—helped drive this specialization. With all its advancements and associated growth, medicine was pushing itself out of homes and the community and into larger, higher tech medical offices, emergency rooms, and hospitals.

My grandfather was a slow adapter. He never lost his black bag. He once quipped, "How easy is it to just have to know *one* organ system? Seems boring." He cherished his role as a generalist and enjoyed the intellectual challenge it presented

In hearing his career stories, I was always struck by two things.

First, he worked incredibly hard. For decades, his daily routine was to see patients in his office all day, often six days per week. Then he'd come home for dinner with the family, which was always a formal, sit-down meal that he and my grandmother would prioritize to ensure it wasn't rushed. These dinners were the foundation of his family time, which he otherwise constantly sacrificed for the sake of patient care. Following dinner, he would retire to his office to finish his day's work—completing charts and making phone calls.

Routinely, in fact the majority of nights, he would finish the day by visiting the homes of his patients he was concerned about.

Back then, especially early in his career, there were far fewer emergency rooms compared to today. If a patient felt bad or had an urgent issue, they would usually first call their physician—typically on their home phone. (This was long before the use of pagers, call services, or HIPAA-secure text apps.) Throughout his career, my grandfather continued the practice of meeting his patients at their homes. He resisted referring them to the emergency rooms popping up in response to urban sprawl, which had made traditional home visits increasingly impractical for most physicians. He simply believed patients did better in the comfort of their own homes, as long as they could be observed carefully (an idea that has recently become much more in vogue).

As a young boy, my father often accompanied my grandfather on his routine late-night house calls, entering the homes by his side. Both of them, I imagine, enjoyed the opportunity to carve out some time together. One of my father's jobs was to carry my grandfather's famous black bag.

The second thing that struck me when he told his stories was how much he *loved* his job. There he was, in his early 90s, reliving his glory days of clinical practice with an excitement and continued scientific fascination that often led him to get lost in his own stories. As I was actively contemplating career choices, his passion for the profession was as good an advertisement as one could hope for. He loved the science of medicine.

In hindsight, he was a complete nerd. He continued to read medical journals until he died.

He loved and appreciated the ability—and the power—of medicine to help those truly in need, to relieve suffering. His stories would prioritize the challenging cases involving patients with severe diseases or living in severe poverty, frequently referencing his work in the Los Angeles Receiving Hospital. He often provided free care for those who could not pay.

The older he got, the more I prioritized my visits with him. During Christmas break of my sophomore year in college, in the middle of my organic chemistry love-fest, I drove up to Santa Barbara for a visit. During one of our typical living room conversations, I shared with him my growing interest in medicine.

His reaction took me by surprise.

———

At the time, in the mid-1990s, medicine was in the middle of one of its many tumultuous periods. Average Americans were becoming increasingly aware of the growing impact of healthcare costs on our country, but more importantly, in their daily lives. When my grandfather started his career, the cost of American healthcare was similar to that of other Western countries, responsible for approximately 5 percent of our national GDP. By the mid-1990s, America had jumped way out into the lead, with healthcare-related spending consuming approximately 13 percent of our national GDP.[1] The financial impact of medicine's high cost was becoming increasingly felt by employers and companies that could not keep up, as they were forced to reduce benefits or salaries in order to continue providing health benefits. However, those most impacted were the working poor—those who didn't qualify for Medicaid but who weren't provided health insurance by their employers. They were left uninsured and susceptible to poor health outcomes and their associated financial consequences. Our nation was left vulnerable to the inevitable healthcare disparities that result from such a two-tiered system.

Medical systems were getting larger and larger, increasingly prioritizing profits over health. Patients who could afford it got the care they needed—and a lot of expensive care they didn't need. Poor, sick patients who really needed medical care were left neglected by health systems that viewed them as financial losses on their balance sheets. The results, on both ends of this spectrum, were expensive—and inefficient.

People were starting to recognize healthcare in the country for what it was becoming—as Warren Buffett would later describe "the tapeworm of American economic competitiveness."[2]

These escalating medical costs resulted in contentious political debates around healthcare transformation efforts, which were designed to help bend this unsustainable cost curve. Bipartisan collaboration and compromise between political parties to implement policies that benefit our country has always been a challenge. However, it's foundational to our political process. When it came to healthcare transformation efforts in the early 1990s, such collaboration would prove to be impossible.

In 1991, over 35 different healthcare reform bills were proposed in Congress. None passed.

President George H. Bush introduced his own reform plan the following year that included lowering unsustainable Medicare costs while expanding healthcare coverage to 35 million uninsured Americans. However, it also didn't pass Congress.

In the 1992 presidential campaign, Bill Clinton ran heavily on healthcare reform and, once in office, sought to make it a cornerstone of his administration. He appointed then-First Lady Hillary Clinton to develop and lead a task force. Perhaps emboldened by a Democratic majority in both chambers of Congress, the task force's National Health Security Plan proved to be much more aggressive than previous reform proposals. It essentially aimed to overhaul healthcare in America. It proposed universal coverage provided through qualified government health plans that could determine fees and impose spending limits. It also included mandates that employers provide health insurance, and regulations of benefit design.[3]

Pushback was intense, driven by insurance and healthcare lobbyists. Even though many couldn't access it, America had developed the most advanced and high-tech healthcare system in the world. It was able to cure the broken in dramatic and effective ways. We were a scientific wonder, the proud result of advancements in medical science that were increasingly impressive and mind-boggling. Could you really put a price on "the impressive and mind-boggling" when it was aimed at improving health and saving lives? The main counterpoint against reform was the potential loss of access to these health options and benefits that Americans had become accustomed to—ignoring the complete lack of access that already existed, mainly along socioeconomic lines, for tens of millions of Americans.

Nobody really could disagree with the problem as stated by Bill Clinton in a 1993 address to Congress: "On any given day, over 37 million Americans—most of them working people and their little children—have no health insurance at all. And in spite of all this, our medical bills are growing at over twice the rate of inflation, and the United States spends over a third more of its income on health care than any other nation on Earth."[4]

However, nobody could agree on how to solve these issues. The risks seemed high. Unlike other industries, failed reform efforts could potentially harm the health of the average American. The aggressive push toward governmental mandates and control proved to be too much for many Americans. Concerns around uniquely un-American regulation of a uniquely American high-tech, expensive, global-leading healthcare system scared off legislators from both sides of the aisle. The Democrats lost collaborative support within their own party. Efforts became fragmented. Eventually, everybody just kind of gave up ... quietly.

Our large, expensive healthcare system seemed already too big and complex for corporate and government attempts to rein it in, even as it increasingly paralyzed our economy. Thus the can was kicked way down the road, and cost trajectories remained firmly pointed in unsustainable directions. The tapeworm continued to feed and grow.

My grandfather had become increasingly focused on these political debates over the years, referencing them in visits with family. But honestly I would tune them out, as they were relatively boring compared to his war and medical stories.

That afternoon, when I started my conversation with him about entering a career in medicine, I had minimal understanding or appreciation for the entire political backdrop. So I had imagined that he would be excited, potentially thrilled, that one of his 19 grandchildren (I was the fourth youngest) had finally decided to follow him into a career that he had clearly loved.

I forget exactly how I told him. I remember it being something relatively lame and straightforward, such as, "I think I want to go into medicine," followed by some rambling about how much I loved my biology courses.

We only have one chance at a reflexive reaction. His was not one of excitement. It was concern.

He had always shown an incredible knack for saying the exact right thing, perfectly, without hesitation in his conversations. This time, he appeared uncharacteristically rattled. He sat quietly for a few seconds, seeming to struggle with his response.

"Medicine is not what it used to be," he said. A few more seconds of silence followed before he added, "It's important to realize, medicine is *not* a career; it is a vocation."

It was clear he did not mean this as an advertisement but a warning—and perhaps, to some extent, a nostalgic wish that he hoped still held some truth. Perhaps he was also nervous about pushing me into a field that no longer resembled the one he loved—a field he'd glamorized through his stories, but which had evolved to become almost unrecognizable since he began his career in the 1930s.

Medicine is not a career; it is a vocation.

I've thought about this last quote often—almost daily—during my career, especially during the rougher days when I see my patients suffer from pathologies I struggle to help them with. I've thought about it as we develop public health models and try to identify the root causes of so many of the current inefficiencies and related poor outcomes in medicine.

My grandfather never really circled back to qualify his comments—to reassure or encourage. He stayed firm with his initial response and reaction, which would be enough to make me second-guess my decision and step off the fast track to medical school applications.

In hindsight, this was probably the best thing that could have happened to me. The two years I took between college and medical school helped shape my own path in medicine. This time allowed me to think and gain perspective. What I perceived as a confusing/mixed message from my grandfather was probably the opposite. Perhaps, true to form, he knew exactly what I needed to hear.

4

THE COSTUME

Four years after that conversation in my grandfather's living room, I stood outside of Georgetown University's Gaston Hall, sweating in a starchy, short white coat in the brutal humidity of a typical Washington, DC, summer day.

I had arrived in DC just two days earlier, my 1989 Honda Civic packed with everything I owned. I liked to procrastinate in life. I was good at it. As such, I found, at the last minute, a group of five other first-year medical students needing one more person to pay rent for a beautiful Georgetown greystone house on a cherry-blossom-tree-lined street two blocks from campus. The only catch: I got the last room available, which was a 9-by-8-foot "bedroom" (pretty sure it was a converted closet) that, instead of wallpaper, inexplicably had green cloth with a weird 1970s pattern on it over its walls. I rushed out and bought a futon and some blankets to complete my "home."

As I baked in the summer heat before entering our white coat ceremony, I was exhausted. I had barely slept in the whirlwind of getting settled over the previous few days. I felt like I was simultaneously collapsing over one finish line while just getting started on the next race, which would undoubtedly be more exhausting—and exciting. I was surrounded by more than 160 students entering their first year of medical school, sweating in the same white, starchy coats that looked more costume-ish than legit-doctor-ish.

The white coat ceremony is a rite of passage signaling the beginning of a medical student's journey. Being there that day was the result of years of successful, hard work. High school success led to success in college and admittance to a medical school that accepted only 3 percent of its more than 10,000 applications annually. Pride and excitement drifted through the air. Many students had family members and friends who came in for the event. For the most part, I think we were all impressed and relieved by how cool our fellow students seemed to be, given that we were about to spend the next four years together. People seemed modest, friendly, and outgoing. There were obviously some outliers—the ones who didn't even have to say a word to reveal their arrogance, or some who decided to go ahead and avoid any doubt by talking.

We spent the next hour in the beautiful Gaston Hall—which added to the event's formality and sense of importance, as deans and faculty gave inspirational talks in the same room that had hosted numerous American and foreign presidents, prime ministers, and heads of state. Most seats, both in the balcony and orchestra section, were occupied.

At the end of the ceremony, we rose as a group to recite the Hippocratic Oath—a common tradition for incoming students in most medical schools. Citing the famous Greek text, new medical students swear an oath to uphold foundational ethical standards in medicine and patient care, including to do "no harm or injustice to them" while developing treatments that would "benefit my patients according to my greatest ability and judgment."[1] I couldn't help but reflect back to the advice—or perhaps more accurately, the warning—my grandfather gave years earlier. In the oath, I recognized his message around *vocation*.

Following the ceremony, many pictures were taken with proud family members and friends. As I had nobody who came in for the ceremony, I joined a small group that left early to walk down to the famous Georgetown bar, The Tombs, to start a celebration that would last late into the night. It was a victory party that honored the road behind us, including our successful navigation to get to that white coat ceremony. We were not necessarily focused on the road ahead of us—its patients, its vocation—or the oath we had just naively sworn to.

5

THE RED PILL

Dr. Jim O'Connell helped to start the Boston Health Care for the Homeless Program after finishing his residency at Massachusetts General Hospital in 1985. Originally it was meant to be a one-year hiatus before he entered a fellowship in hematology/oncology. Almost 40 years later, he is still on that hiatus, having built the largest healthcare for the homeless program in the nation while helping to develop national policies and clinical best practices around the medical treatment of vulnerable populations.

After graduating salutatorian at Notre Dame, Jim spent time wandering the world, picking up a degree in theology and philosophy from Cambridge University in England, teaching high school in Hawaii for a bit, and then kind of *hippying* it up for years on a farm in Vermont before strolling into Harvard Medical School. As brilliant as he is kindhearted, he was a perfect pioneer for developing a new field of medicine focused on caring for those suffering from homelessness. Simultaneously, his program would challenge broader systemic inefficiencies around how medicine has historically treated the poor.

Jim built BHCHP from scratch—in soup kitchens, homeless shelters, and on the street, knocking down constant barriers as he did so. His story was documented in an incredible book by Tracy Kidder, *Rough Sleepers*, published in 2023, which provides insight into his work and the patients he has served.

I stumbled into BHCHP by accident while trying to avoid moving to Alaska.

In medical school, I received a National Health Service Corp (NHSC) scholarship that paid for my medical education at Georgetown. In return, after completing my training, I was committed to practicing primary care in a designated area of need. The goal was to help address a primary care shortage in our nation that disproportionately impacts certain regions and communities.

When it was time to fulfill my NHSC obligations upon completing my chief residency year in Chicago, eight years of training after I'd first donned my starchy white coat in the thick Georgetown humidity, my wife and I scanned the list of potential physician placements. The list that year was typical for the program, filled with many opportunities in some pretty interesting places across the country. Aside from one spot in Saint Croix, a position we discovered didn't ultimately exist, most locations were isolated and not necessarily very appealing to the average person. But that was kind of the whole idea of the program—to get primary care physicians to places nobody else would go.

I was initially excited about an opening in Unalaska—a fishing community on the distant tip of the islands jetting off from southern Alaska. It was essentially a rock in the Pacific, known for its treeless yet still beautiful landscape. My wife, Colleen, told me she would divorce me before actually going there. I thought she was kidding. She assured me she was not.

One day, we noticed a position that had opened up at Boston's Health Care for the Homeless. While the location was awesome—and Colleen was happy to return to New England, as she was originally from Granby, Connecticut—I was hesitant. I'd envisioned fulfilling my NHSC obligation working in a community of people who really needed help—people who "wanted to help themselves" and would be engaged with their healthcare. I would strut in with my abundant medical knowledge to help deliver that desperately needed, and wanted, care—very *Northern Exposure*-ish (which would have made Unalaska a perfect setting). At the time, so many of the health issues related to homelessness seemed self-inflicted to me. How could I possibly help patients who didn't want to help themselves?

The location was too good to pass up, however, so I flew out from Chicago to interview. I was blown away.

I met with Jim in his crowded, relatively messy office with the noise of South Boston's Mass Avenue humming in the background. Actually, there was no *relative* about it—it was *definitively* messy. In his defense, I supposed that genius was hard to keep tidy.

I think anybody who has met Jim O'Connell would agree that there are a few things that strike you right away.

First, he is brilliant. A quick glance at his resume will clearly reveal this.

Second, he has the best heart of anybody you will ever meet—which no doubt is helpful, in fact necessary, to keep pushing through the relentless pioneering work he has led for the past 40 years. The stamina needed to persevere through the pain and hardship he has had to witness in his patients throughout his career requires a determined heart.

Lastly, he is pathologically humble—legit humility, not false, superficial self-deprecation. He is deft in quickly deflecting any attention or praise, typically directing it right back to his patients who he serves and admires.

He possesses this "triple threat" of sainthood: brilliance, kindness, and humility.

Hearing about his vision, perspectives, and interactions with patients experiencing homelessness was fascinating—it instantly exposed and challenged my personal stereotypes. As we sat in his crowded office in the spring of 2007, he appeared to downplay the incredible clinical model he had pioneered to reduce the suffering of the most challenging patients in Boston. He knew better than anybody it was a difficult system to work in. Decades earlier, when he made this career decision, he could not have anticipated the amount of personal and professional sacrifice that would be required. Early in his career, Jim easily pushed into 100-plus-hour work weeks (pause to think about that), as he knew if he didn't, there would be nobody else to help his patients. It was often literally a matter of life and death—which was a hell of a responsibility.

While he remained fully invested despite the personal sacrifices he made throughout his career, he was cautious not to oversell healthcare for the homeless to young, perhaps overly idealistic physicians as they entered into their own careers. Oncologists, for example, would make a whole lot more than public health providers—and probably enjoy a more steady work-life balance.

Research, however, has demonstrated that despair isn't necessarily related to a lack of happiness but rather a lack of meaning and purpose in life. As renowned psychologist Martin Seligman wrote: "Meaning comes from belonging to and serving something beyond yourself and from developing the best within you."[1]

Cranking out the hours in a medical system with misdirected priorities can suck out one's meaning and purpose. It can lead to despair. There's a reason why physician burnout has skyrocketed over the past few generations, driving its providers away from a field they once were excited to enter.

Nothing triggers burnout more than loss of purpose.

Making sacrifices in our personal lives, especially around friends or family, is perhaps more acceptable in the context of vocation than with just a "job"—especially one that forces providers to practice contrary to the vocational aspects they once swore to uphold and found inspirational.

That day in his crowded and noisy office, Jim worked hard to subtly caution me, but he did a horrible job at it. He had purpose. He couldn't disguise this, nor the ultimate passion and love he felt for his patients—and, therefore, his job. He'd sacrificed so much in his life with those long hours, late nights, and busy weekends. But, ultimately, I don't think he would have changed a thing. He'd built a whole team—an entire program—on this foundation of passion and purpose. This was a noticeable contrast to what I had seen in most physicians during my medical training.

I was sold after my visit with Jim and the program. I still felt burdened and hesitant by my stereotypes of homelessness, but the model, its purpose, and the team battling to implement it ultimately made my decision a no-brainer. I saw something unique and fascinating in the model and wanted to be part of it.

A few days later, I excitedly accepted the offer during a phone call with BHCHP's medical director, Dr. Greg Wagoner. However, he didn't reflexively reciprocate my excitement.

"You realize, Brian, homeless medicine is really its own specialty," he responded in a cautious tone that mirrored Jim's. It almost felt like a scene from *The Matrix*, with Morpheus warning Neo about the implications of taking the red pill versus the blue pill. I was being warned about the potential burdens of selecting a path that would result in learning and confronting realities that might be inconvenient and resisted by the larger healthcare system we still must function within ... about going down a path that challenged a system that might not want to be challenged ... and the potential personal impact of doing so.

To their credit, everybody was working to make sure I was going into the field of homeless medicine with eyes wide open—which, despite their best efforts, they failed to do. I chose to misinterpret Dr. Wagoner's message more as an advertisement than a warning. I was excited, obliviously naïve, and still married after deciding not to move to Unalaska. In my defense, it's impossible to truly understand the downstream consequences of life decisions you're making in your late 20s—the financial implications, their impact on work-life balance, and the potential for burnout. Also, when you're young, the more somebody warns you about something, the cooler it seems.

Years later, however, I feel a similar sense of obligation not to oversell our field to young residents and students who may still be "blinded" by the idealism of youth. Although I'm increasingly realizing that perhaps it's all semantics. Perhaps we, as we advance in our career, are the ones who get "blinded" by age?

6

WHY?

I was hired into a new position within Boston Health Care for the Homeless that was designed to be part of a pilot "integrated care model." At the time, in 2007, I had never heard of an integrated care model. The basic idea is to have teams of medical *and* behavioral health providers working side-by-side to provide comprehensive care to patients. The model recognizes that medical conditions are often complicated, or even driven, by mental health conditions—and vice versa. To effectively treat one, you must simultaneously address the other. This is especially true in very sick patients. Mental and physical health are unequivocally linked. Our failure to historically recognize and adequately address this in medicine has been the source of a lot of our costly, and deadly, historic inefficiencies.

When I started BHCHP, I didn't even grasp this at the broader conceptual level, much less the more complex yet ultimately more intuitive physiologic one that I will discuss later in the book.

By this time in my career, I'd had very little training in mental illness. We'd had a few weeks of classroom work in our second year of medical school and a three-week rotation in my third year that involved a scarring experience in a crowded, poorly staffed, and depressing inpatient facility. This lack of exposure to psychiatry continued into my residency. I therefore entered BHCHP with little experience or knowledge about what would prove to be foundational to the care models we were to develop. Honestly, my views on mental health at the time were likely more driven by common societal stereotypes and misunderstandings than by medical knowledge.

Our team was a sort of "integrated care model on steroids." Besides two nurse practitioners and me, the team had a psychiatrist, a case manager, and a respite care floor nurse. The model was designed around teams that would work in both of the primary clinical settings of BHCHP: the outpatient clinics operating out of hospitals and local homeless shelters, and the program's 100-plus-bed medical respite facility.

Medical respite is a model designed to help homeless patients who are too sick to be on the streets or shelters but too healthy to be in the hospital. After an illness, most of us don't leave the hospital doing backflips, dishing out high fives, and feeling back to normal. If we have pneumonia or suffered from a heart attack or case of pancreatitis, we go home from the hospital and take additional time to rest as our bodies continue healing. We're stable enough not to require hospital beds meant for our most critically ill patients but not yet recovered enough to hop right back into our normal lives.

Unhoused populations don't have this luxury of a stable place to rest and continue recovering. For patients without secure housing, this often results in a quick and dangerous deterioration upon discharge, leading to frequent readmissions back into the hospital.

Historically, BHCHP's medical and behavioral health providers would work in only one of the two settings. By spanning across both, the program hoped to improve continuity of care for patients while allowing their providers to develop stronger clinical relationships with sicker patients who were often in the respite facility.

Our integrated care team's first meeting was very informal. The new team met in the much tidier office of Dr. Monica Bharel, the then-medical director of our respite program, who was the innovator of the model we were implementing. She, unlike Dr. O'Connell and Dr. Wagoner, was incapable of even trying to dampen the joy and excitement for her work. She had no interest in doing so. It radiated from her—contagious and motivating—and was the hallmark of her successful career, which would eventually include becoming the Secretary of Health of Massachusetts.

All of us on the team were relatively young, early in our careers, and excited to get started. The other two medical providers, Carolyn Abbanat and Kathleen Saunders, had worked as nurse practitioners for the previous few years in the respite care center. Kathy George was the floor nurse, beloved by patients who would frequent our respite care program. James Noonan, with his incredible, curly red hair, was our case manager and a relatively non-obnoxious Boston College grad. He would later go back to school and return to the program as a medical provider.

I was the only new person on the team, besides the psychiatrist who couldn't make it to the meeting that day. But when I heard her name, I was thrilled—Dr. Shunda McGahee, an old former Georgetown Medical School classmate of mine. She was brilliant, outgoing, and would light up any room she was in. She was famous for her Georgetown Medical School Talent Show comedy skits. I had not seen or talked to her since medical school and had no idea she was even in Boston until that meeting. I was beyond excited to get started.

A few weeks later, I saw my first patient with Carolyn in our respite care center. Kenneth suffered from schizophrenia and a severe case of venous insufficiency in his legs with associated ulcers. He'd come into the respite facility after his ulcers had deteriorated and become infected.

He was tall and emaciated, making his leg swelling appear even more pronounced. Being mid-summer, his extreme tan reflected that he didn't use shelters and spent almost all his time outside. He had a thick beard and long hair, oily and unkempt. Even though he'd been admitted the day before we saw him, it was clear he had not showered yet—nor had he likely done so for months. The staff was working on it.

Kenneth loudly barged into the exam room to start our visit, irritated that the nurse had awoken him. I could see his leg bandages were soaked with a yellowish/greenish discharge. They didn't smell great. As he sat, quiet and frustrated, I broke into my line of questioning, almost instinctively.

He, almost instinctively, wanted no part of it. He didn't answer any of my clinical questions but instead kept voicing frustration that I was even asking them. I was immediately hitting a brick wall—on my first patient—which I defensively attributed to a likely antisocial personality disorder that had not yet been diagnosed. He was clearly displaying the "socially difficult" criteria of the disorder. I pushed on, futilely, for a few more awkward minutes until Carolyn jumped in to save me.

Kenneth was relatively new to the program, so Carolyn didn't know him either. She asked about his accent and where he was from (Mississippi). She asked about his previous medical and treatment interactions. Within a few minutes, his defenses seemed to drop enough that he started to answer some of her questions, albeit still begrudgingly. He eventually allowed us to take down his dressings, which revealed some macerated, somewhat infected, and definitely malodorous leg wounds. Carolyn even got him to crack a smile. As he became more comfortable and conversational, I felt increasingly guilty about my reflexive and ultimately inaccurate antisocial personality disorder diagnosis from minutes earlier.

He was already on the correct oral antibiotic. Carolyn turned to ask for my thoughts on wound care, although she clearly knew the answer—almost an obligatory and courteous but not well-disguised "ask the doctor" routine.

"What kind of wound dressing do you want to use?"

I was paralyzed, stumped—on my very first clinical question as a doctor for the program. I realized suddenly that throughout my entire medical training, I'd had literally no education on wound care. None. I couldn't even talk the language to fake it. I sat silent for a few seconds before my futile attempt to save face: "What do *you* think?" My smile made it blatantly obvious that I had no clue.

She nicely put me out of my misery, answering with what she already knew would be the best option for him: "Xeroform, with non-adherent gauze and kerlix ... with overlying compression," or something like that.

I nodded approval; she had said it with such confidence, I just guessed she must be right. If that patient had presented with septic shock and needed to be managed with a ventilator, I could have nailed it and impressed everybody with my textbook management after my four years of residency training. But he didn't need a ventilator. He needed "Xeroform," and I didn't even recognize that word.

The entire interaction—with my very first patient—instantly humbled me, making me realize I must immediately shift back into the learning mode I thought I'd graduated out of.

I've been stuck there ever since.

That night, I went home to Google "Xeroform"—and to study up on the clinical diagnosis of patients with antisocial personality disorders.

Every Wednesday morning at BHCHP, our team would pile into an exam room at our respite care center and see the 13 patients on our team census. It was always crowded. It was always awesome.

We would ask our patients how they were doing, review their chart for events over the past week, and discuss their medical plan. Seeing so many people genuinely focused on what was best for them was therapeutic for the patient. It also helped that, given the personalities on our team, the meetings involved a lot of laughing and joking.

Laughter, undoubtedly, is one of the best medicines we have. It can very much put people at ease—when used correctly. In its own way, it can also provide some dignity—a common way to relate on a human level. We may take humor for granted in our daily interactions, but it's often nonexistent in the lives of individuals experiencing homelessness.

Our integrated care team was, admittedly, a very resource-rich model. It felt like we were throwing the kitchen sink at these cases, with the number of providers and staff dedicated to patient care. However, given the high medical costs of many of these patients, which routinely went into the six figures, improved outcomes could easily result in a cost savings that still dwarfed the staffing cost of the model. It was much cheaper to manage these patients with a team in respite care rather than one in the ICU, which is where many of our patients, including those with developing infections of venous stasis ulcers, were headed if not for our interventions.

We developed a "panel" of patients assigned to our team over time. We'd follow them when they came in for respite care and in the outpatient settings as well. Our team worked out of two of our medical clinics—our main one downtown at Boston Medical Center and a satellite clinic in the homeless shelter on South Boston's Long Island.

Located in the middle of the Boston Harbor, the island had a fascinating history that dated back to Native Americans and served as a strategic military location for all of our nation's early wars. In the 1900s, it was designated to be used for social services—serving the city's poor, sick, and addicted. It also served as a homeless shelter. Each night, hundreds of homeless residents would wait in long lines in South Boston to hop on buses and make the 30-minute trip to the shelter (often much longer if traffic on 93 South was bad). Early the next morning, shelter guests would have to get back on the buses to return to the city.

Access to the island was restricted to the public. To get from the mainland onto the island, cars and buses had to drive over a dilapidated, two-lane steel bridge. Police were stationed on each end to control traffic to ensure no more than a few vehicles were on it at a time, so the bridge wouldn't collapse into the water. One of the BCHCHP nurses gave me a "survival kit" when I first started there —which included a hammer, swim goggles, and a snorkel. I kept it in my car all four years. The bridge was eventually demolished in 2015.

While some people were opposed to the idea of "shipping out" hundreds of unhoused individuals each night—as a type of concession to the not-in-my-backyard (NIMBY) arguments of communities that were blocking additional local shelters—once the guests got to Long Island, many found the setting peaceful. The shelter itself was typical: crowded and stacked with bunks. The open landscape of the island, however, and its location on the north end of the island—which facilitated views of incredible sunsets over the harbor with Boston's skyline in the background—helped to provide a calm and therapeutic contrast to the stress and chaos they experienced in the city during the day.

In the winter, it would already be getting dark by the time I'd arrive for my 4 to 8 p.m. clinical shift. A family of raccoons would meet us almost nightly in the parking lot; they became "friendly" with many of the regular guests who would often feed them, but they were also responsible for the only raccoon bites I've treated in my career.

Long Island was a "wet shelter," allowing people to be intoxicated as long as they weren't disruptive or dangerous. When bad things did happen, it would take a while for ambulances from "the mainland" to make the trek all the way to the island, over the dilapidated bridge—as I learned while managing a patient with status epilepticus (persistent seizure) for over an hour during a New Year's Eve snowstorm.

This team model allowed us to better establish trust through a continuity of care across settings. This was key, since clinical trust is everything—a prerequisite to any successful clinical interaction between patient and provider.

In patients with historically poor experiences with their healthcare providers, trust can be hard to develop. But in the quiet of the respite care center, away from the chaos of the streets, we had a unique opportunity to develop, often slowly, these relationships. It could take days, even weeks, as with Kenneth, our patient with leg ulcers, who we ultimately followed for years. However, once a patient trusted us, we could leverage that trust to improve medical outcomes through continuity of care—whether through stabilizing them at respite, seeing them in the hospital, or treating their raccoon bites or seizures at Long Island. Patients felt known, not abandoned.

This model also allowed for a greater clinical benefit per patient during the respite stay, as we could focus not only on the acute issues leading to the admission but also on effectively addressing preventive care and chronic disease management issues that may have been hard to address in the outpatient setting. We had a captive audience who we knew well. For example, if a 52-year-old, female patient recently diagnosed with diabetes was admitted to the medical respite care program to recover from gallbladder surgery, during her stay, we could administer her influenza and pneumonia vaccines, get her mammogram screening up-to-date, and initiate her on a diabetic medication while monitoring for side effects. All while she improved from the surgery.

It didn't take long before I started to better appreciate the benefits of our model's integrated care aspect, including the need to work with Dr. McGahee to address the behavioral health issues or our case manager, James, to address the social issues that were driving the complicated medical issues we were attempting to treat. This need to address both physical and mental health was a lesson we would try to teach the residents and students who trained with us at the respite center, in our clinics, or in the hospital.

Resident teaching conferences usually involved presenting a complex patient for group discussions around diagnosis and treatment. We typically presented this as a "what is wrong with this patient?" riddle followed by education on the identified pathologies after diagnosis and problem-solving by the group. Part of this exercise included working through the differential diagnoses—a list of possible medical explanations for the presenting symptoms. The goal was to understand what led to the patient's situation and decide what was "the next best thing" we could do to maximize their outcome.

That's really what medicine is all about: working with the patient every step of the way to determine, based on what we currently know, the next best step for them and their health.

One of the cases presented came from one of my inpatient weeks attending at Boston Medical Center. This patient suffered from homelessness, addiction, severe anxiety, and type 2 diabetes. She presented in septic shock with an infected diabetic foot ulcer. After the case was presented at a morning report conference, I asked the residents to "list everything going on with this patient." Per usual, they reported her most urgent issues first, those that needed immediate stabilization. They then worked backwards.

They listed septic shock first. This was life-threatening, but it was often treatable with "goal-directed therapy" that involved stabilizing the patient by fighting the infection with antibiotics while stabilizing low blood pressure with IV fluids and medications.

They then moved on to the foot ulcer—the source of the infection. They suggested they would need a surgical consult to see if the wound needed to be cleaned and debrided—or did the foot need to be amputated?

Diabetes was next on the list. Her diabetes was not only the underlying cause of the foot ulcer, but it was also complicating its current treatment, as she presented with acutely high blood sugars. Infection loves high blood sugars, which meant her glucose would need to be better controlled in order to optimize outcomes.

The residents then moved on to her addiction. Having suffered from chronic alcoholism, the patient was demonstrating symptoms of physiological withdrawals on presentation. This would need to be addressed per "CIWA protocol" (Clinical Institute Withdrawal Assessment for Alcohol), where patients are provided medications to help them safely taper off the alcohol to avoid the potentially life-threatening symptoms of withdrawals.

These problems were enough to keep the treatment team busy. And if the septic shock, infected foot, high blood sugars, and alcohol withdrawal were adequately addressed in the short-term, the patient would have a good chance of surviving. But the team stopped there.

"Anything else?" I asked. They looked around and shrugged their shoulders. They felt pretty good about the list.

Why is the patient septic? *Because of the infected ulcer.*

Why did the patient have an ulcer? *Because of the decreased sensation in her feet related to the diabetic damage.*

Why did it get infected? *Because of poor hygiene and high blood sugars.*

Why did the patient have really high blood sugars? *Because she didn't have access to insulin.*

Why did the patient not have access to insulin? *Because she was homeless, living outside, and without a refrigerator.*

Why was the patient homeless? This is where it started to get a bit more confusing and less concrete. *Social dysfunction related to alcoholism? To anxiety? To something else?*

Why was the person anxious? Why did the patient suffer from addiction? Why … why … why?

As questions with definitive answers—based on knowledge and associated learned algorithms—evolve "upstream" to more challenging ones we are less certain about, we become fatigued. To prevent exhaustion and stay functional, we as medical providers stay in the familiar, with our established algorithms and protocols—even if that means we're really only treating symptoms. We fix, and bill (expensively), and then send the patient back out. We provide perfect examples of Einstein's (although some debate its attribution to him) definition of *insanity*, "doing the same thing over and over again and expecting different results," until one day, the patient gets there too late for early goal-directed therapy or any of other interventions that might save them. The sepsis wins. The patient, quickly forgotten, becomes just one more data point reinforcing statistics around poor outcomes and early mortality. We shrug off our ignorance and keep working in the familiarity of the downstream.

Turning around and pushing upstream is hard, so we just stop asking why and fail to reverse-engineer the problems our patients battle. We don't get far enough upstream to find the true root causes; often, we do not even come close.

We need to keep pushing upstream. We must keep asking why. This was the message I would constantly attempt to get across to young residents and students. *Keep trying to identify—so we can treat—root causes. We can't commit the cardinal sin of medicine: treating symptoms instead of underlying etiologies of disease.*

Yet as I loudly preached, I failed to realize I was doing the very thing I was warning them about.

I remained largely ignorant of my own ignorance.

In my defense, this wasn't the first time this had happened in medicine.

Knowledge of mechanism is everything.

Our team-based integrated care model worked well and was subsequently adopted throughout BHCHP. Our team was young. We were all relatively early in our careers. We were battling the most challenging and aggressive cases, but doing so as a team. And we were still idealistic and energetic enough to have fun while we were doing it, supported by leadership and the veteran providers we were learning from.

This was by design. Jim and the BHCHP leadership had intentionally built their program in a way to prevent burnout. Manageable patient panels. Quality over quantity. Diversification of roles and clinical sites. And a weekly organization-wide meeting that created a very supportive environment. Jim developed the program to make careers in homeless medicine sustainable. He was deliberate in avoiding the more typical revolving door models of community health centers where patients are left feeling continuously passed around and abandoned, their care scattered. Models where providers are expected to see unrealistic numbers of patients each day, despite being asked to manage the sickest, poorest, and most complicated residents in a community.

This was the norm in many of the NHSC health clinics that I interviewed with prior to coming to BHCHP. These clinics were focused on year-to-year numbers that involved a pretty obvious strategy of bringing in young, energetic, hopefully-idealistic new doctors and burning them out with large volumes and sick patients —eventually stifling that idealism after a few years ... before bringing in the next crew. With their idealism crushed, the young providers would leave with a clinical PTSD from their experience that would lead them to avoid public health moving forward in their careers.

The field of homeless medicine, with its steep learning curves, needs the leadership and experience of weathered veteran providers. This is especially true in a field where the *science of medicine* is not nearly as important as the *art of medicine*, where more knowledge is gained through experience than textbooks. The field needs consistency. Provider burnout in such a challenging model of care is almost inevitable if you don't protect against it, and this can stall advancements and progress.

The foundation of the BHCHP model was to protect against this burnout. BCHCP had an excellent balance of veteran, knowledgeable providers providing mentorship to energetic, idealistic younger providers. In fact, when I left after four years, I was truly an anomaly.

———

The best leaders in medicine—and across all industries, I imagine—are those who are humble enough to continuously learn and improve. They can identify what their teams do well and do it better as well as what they don't do well and do it *much* better. They turn weaknesses into strengths. But it all starts with an honest humility to admit when they aren't good at something.

In medicine, we are good at a lot of things; unfortunately, humility is not one of them.

It takes patience, determination, brilliance, and perhaps even some courage to push and challenge a system that doesn't want to be challenged or admit its weakness. I found the approach the BHCHP leaders used with the local health systems to be brilliant and strategic. If they pushed too hard against resistance, they would likely reflexively be told to screw off. Instead, they had to engage the systems and demonstrate the intuitive—that there is both a humanistic and a financial return on investment in efficiently managing sick populations—in a way that made it speak for itself.

Most healthcare leadership and administration teams are

inevitably swallowed into a system we know is fundamentally broken. Systems that recruit and hire administrative leadership will likely prioritize their continued financial success and existence above all else, inefficiencies and all. Intelligent and good people get caught up with these entrenched priorities and associated large salaries. They are hired to help *lead*, not necessarily to help *change*—to demonstrate and highlight success, not to admit to weaknesses.

When you're dealing with public health, you're out in the community, not protected by the walls of medical silos and their payment structures. You have a front-row seat to the impact of these current healthcare inefficiencies—on actual patients. You see the cost and suffering. You see the death. For these reasons, some of the best medical leaders in terms of innovation and change advocacy come from the world of public health. These leaders are more empowered to go against the grain and more aware of why it's necessary. Yet historically, these public health leaders have been ignored by larger systems not incentivized to listen to their stories or advocacy as they continue to profit handsomely on the receiving end of the expensive brokenness.

BHCHP leadership was able to strategically engage large health systems. They were able to humanize their historically marginalized patients and demonstrate the financial cost of their poor health to the systems, as well as to all levels of government—from city through federal. They got people to understand ... and therefore care ... and therefore engage. It was genius.

I realized at the time, and even more in hindsight, how fortunate I was *on a personal level* to be exposed to this incredible leadership so early in my career. The supportive culture of BHCHP was almost a necessity to ensure I didn't run the other way. My world instantly turned upside down when I realized that my training hadn't empowered me to stroll into BHCHP as an expert, or even really competent—which was incredibly humbling. Even though I was building upon the foundation of my training and education, it felt a lot like starting from scratch. I had to learn rather than teach, follow rather than lead–or perhaps, as they taught me, lead *by* following. I needed to change my mindset to learn how to think differently.

Luckily, their incredible and experienced medical leadership guided me through this process and placed me as securely as possible on an otherwise chaotic career path of public health.

I've been fortunate to continue benefiting from this type of uniquely mission-driven leadership as I've advanced in my career.

7

INVISIBLE

I met Joanne Guarino in my first year at BCHCP. At the time, our respite care center was still located in Jamaica Plain—a building that would later be converted to housing units named after the late Stacy Fitzpatrick, a longtime nurse practitioner at BHCHP. Stacy was an incredible, kindhearted clinician with likely one of the best bedside manners I have ever seen.

I was, in fact, talking with Stacy one morning at the nursing station when, from down the hall, a thick Boston-accented voice bellowed out, "Hey, Dr. Dude—I'll see you in here. Ten minutes." I looked to see the woman who was yelling, pointing to an exam room right next to her. I had never seen her before. I was confused, as I was not sure who she was talking to. I think she saw my confusion, so she decided to clarify. "Ten minutes ... in here!" She said it in a friendly tone, with a subtle smile and a small laugh, but I still definitely made sure I was there 10 minutes later. It just seemed like I should probably do what she said.

Joanne had been admitted to the respite facility the day before to recover from a leg wound. She was assigned to our care team.

The first thing that struck me about Joanne was her overall presence: engaging and gregarious. She very well might have been the most instantly-likeable person I had ever met. There was a glaring contrast between her current social and medical situations and the optimism and happiness she displayed. In her mid-50s, she had experienced more than a lifetime of suffering through emotional and physical trauma. As I learned more about her history over the following weeks while caring for her in respite, this contrast only grew more apparent. Joanne's optimism was contagious, and her resilience both inspiring and fascinating.

She spent her days in respite socializing and encouraging other patients around her. Not at all presumptions or intruding, she waited until they came to her. And they sought her out. From her seat in the group room, she acted as a combination of friend, therapist, and health coach—to the point that I sometimes forgot she was a patient. Her nurturing of others wasn't forced or occupational. It was genuine, which is why it was so successful.

Many of the younger patients saw her as a maternal figure that they had never had. Her attitude was uplifting, while her concern was therapeutic. She related to others through shared experiences that we as providers didn't have. People intuitively trusted her, as she inspired them to keep fighting, to not give up. Often, that alone could be the difference between life and death with our patients.

Joanne did well during her stay.

I would subsequently become Joanne's primary care provider for my next four years in Boston. Given the number and severity of her medical conditions, we would visit every other week in our main outpatient clinic, on Tuesday mornings. She was always my first patient of the day—and the highlight of my week. She provided constant insights and education to a young physician who was fascinated, but often lost and confused, by the field of homeless medicine that I'd stumbled into. She also provided humor. She was hilarious. On more than a few occasions, we got reprimanded by clinic staff for being too loud or disruptive. I would just blame her.

Joanne eventually moved into her own apartment during my second year in Boston. She remained housed from that day forward. The first thing she did upon getting out of the nightmare of homelessness was to rush right back in to help others do the same. Joanne didn't hide from the darkness. She consciously chose to stay in it, determined to provide a light to others through hope and love (and laughter). In doing so, she offered one of the greatest displays of unselfish love I have ever seen.

Over the years, she became an advocate for the unhoused, challenging common stereotypes and misconceptions. She served on the BHCHP's community advisory board as well as the National Consumer Advisory Board (NCAB), a standing committee of the National Health Care for the Homeless Council. In 2015, she authored a book, *Housing Guide: Tips and Tools for a Successful Housing Experience*, to help people moving into housing for the first time.

Years later, I would return to Boston to join Joanne as well as Jim O'Connell in giving a talk about the foundational aspects of the patient-physician relationship in medicine as part of the White Coat ceremonies for Harvard Medical School. They had both been there the previous year and were asked to return. They invited me to tag along. Just like my own ceremony at Georgetown over a decade earlier, it was a very formal affair—in a historic lecture hall decorated with large, very formal oil paintings of famous, brilliant-looking Harvard doctors.

Joanne was an amazing public speaker, and despite the challenging topics she often spoke about, she rarely got nervous. However, this was a large crowd in a very formal setting. I could sense she was anxious when she showed up that afternoon with her two sisters. This was only made worse when a dean of the medical school sought us out to give some well-intended guidance around maintaining the formality of the event, which included having Joanne refer to me as *Doctor* Klausner.

I could see her face drop right away. She had called me many things over the years—Brian, Dude, and a lot of often profanity-laced (but affectionate, I think ... at least that is what I told myself) names, but never *Doctor* Klausner. The increase in her anxiety was noticeable—not that she had any issues simply calling me Doctor Klausner. It was likely more that the request, and the entire setting, were designed around an intentional and deliberate formality that wasn't in her comfort zone.

With a large group of students and faculty filing in, I was getting increasingly nervous for her. Telling her story of trauma and hardships—to give an insight into the nightmare of chronic homelessness—was something she had always made look easy in her talks. But it obviously was not. It was borderline impossible and potentially retriggering. But with her unique strength, resilience, and insight, she had always done an incredible job with it.

Fortunately, realizing the crowd would be large after her experience from the year before, she had prepared by writing some of her thoughts, which gave her some reassurance.

Jim spoke first and gave a typical, awesome Jim speech.

I went up next to introduce Joanne after giving some advice for the students, including a few insights into the importance of the physician-patient relationship.

As Joanne started her talk, my initial concerns were confirmed. I'd never seen her rattled—but she was rattled. Trauma had left her blind in one eye. She struggled to read what she had written out in advance. I could see her hand shaking as she held the paper and tried to work through it. Her voice trembled a bit. After a few minutes, Joanne stopped. She quietly looked up, paused, and blurted out something that I have reminded her of numerous times since it was definitely *not* compliant with the formality request of the dean.

"Fuck it," she said as she put down her notes. A few seconds of awkward silence followed, along with some scattered nervous laughter from the crowd. She definitely had their attention.

What followed was an ad-libbed speech that was probably one of the most genuine and heartfelt—and important—those students had ever heard. It was brilliant, containing many of the common-sense, non-formal, additional profanity-laden insights that she had shared with me over the years. The crowd laughed a lot. And cried. She articulated a message about recognizing the humanity of the patient and utilizing this in our clinical interactions. I hope the audience remembers this throughout their careers.

She returned to speak as part of Harvard's White Coat Ceremony every year after that. And she became a natural. In fact, Harvard's business school has even started to have her present to their students as well. In the book *Rough Sleepers*, Tracy Kidder wrote about one of her White Coat Ceremony talks a few years later. She spoke of the need to be humble. The need to listen. The need to understand. She ended it by summarizing her message with the following advice: "Just not being shithead doctors, you know?" There very well may be no greater message for those entering our profession than this.

Joanne and I would give another talk eight years later when she came down to North Carolina to visit me and my family, who had grown to adore her as an incredible role model. Her trip was a favor to me to provide her insights into homelessness to our state health department leaders to assist with our local advocacy. Also, it was just a good excuse to visit and catch up.

While here, she agreed to talk at a local grade school. This time, the speech was much less formal, replacing the setting of an oil-painting-adorned Harvard Medical School auditorium with a large gym-ish-smelling school gym. Our audience was a few hundred elementary school kids. No profanity this time. Although she did randomly go on an extremely unnecessary tangent about my lack of style when I was in Boston.

This was the deal: In 2008, I was fortunate enough to go to Costco during an incredible sale on some pretty fashionable clothing items. I stocked my entire wardrobe, buying about 10 different patterns of the same shirt and four pairs of the same pants in different colors. If she were as honest and genuine as she had been at her Harvard talk, she would have admitted that the shirts and pants were actually stylish—practical yet not over the top. The shirts were striped. Most of them had really, really nice stripes. That's all I basically wore for my remaining time in Boston. For whatever reason that day, she decided to share this with the kids. "Everybody used to call him Dr. K. I just called him Dr. K-*mart*." Everybody laughed. She thought she was hilarious. I immediately pointed out to everybody that it did not even make sense; the clothes were from *Costco*. But neither she nor the kids cared.

Aside from the inexplicable wardrobe-shaming, she gave another incredible speech that day in the school gym. She shared timeless messages that are as important for school kids as they are for new medical students; in fact, they're important for anybody. She spoke of listening, love, and honoring the humanity of those around us—instead of selfishly discarding them.

At the end of that presentation, a young girl raised her hand.

"What was the most challenging part of experiencing homelessness?" the student inquired.

Joanne replied without hesitation.

"The hardest part was not feeling hungry or cold, or not knowing where I would sleep, but rather feeling *invisible* to others. Sometimes people would not even look at me, even if I was hurt … as if I wasn't even human."

There is nothing more beautiful than human resilience. It is a tragedy when we are blind to it.

8

THE TAPEWORM

In 2010, the Institute of Medicine (IOM) released a report, "The Healthcare Imperative: Lowering Costs and Improving Outcomes."[1] At the time, I was in my fourth year at Boston Health Care for the Homeless, serving as medical director of our Boston Medical Center affiliated outpatient clinic.

The report was released in the early days of a movement in primary care involving the Patient-Centered Medical Home (PCMH) model, which had originated years earlier in pediatrics. The model was built around "primary care that is patient-centered, comprehensive, team-based, coordinated, accessible, and focused on quality and safety."[2]

The model emphasized the potential role and benefits of primary care serving as the foundation (the "home") and the logistical quarterback of patient care, especially when managing chronic disease and optimizing preventive care. As various PCMH pilots and demonstrations nationally resulted in improved clinical outcomes and potential cost savings,[3] this model of care gained more attention from the government, health plans, and employers eager to control escalating medical costs (and, yes, improve patient care). Incentivized by both the potential for clinical quality improvement and the associated financial reimbursements, primary care practices nationwide began to "transform" into medical homes and work through the associated accreditation processes. The entire movement represented an early pivot in how we thought about medical care and, possibly, how we reimbursed it.

We first looked at the PCMH model at BHCHP in 2010. It made sense first to start implementation at our Boston Medical Center outpatient clinic, as it was the largest in our program. When we examined the underlying criteria, our first reaction was, "Aren't we already doing this?" Out of necessity for the patient population we served, BHCHP, since its origins, had prioritized accessibility and centered its care around patients in a comprehensive and coordinated way in the community. We would need to make tweaks and clinical changes to satisfy accreditation requirements, but overall we believed PCMH accreditation made sense for BHCHP and was consistent with our clinical approaches. We were excited to support the larger efforts around this intuitive care model and hopeful it could strengthen primary care while addressing some of the expensive fragmentation that confused patients and led to poor outcomes nationally. We began our efforts that eventually would result in BHCHP successfully becoming a "Level 3" Patient Center Medical Home, the highest recognition a clinic could receive.

These patient-centered medical home models were early attempts by insurance companies and payers to help rein in the costs of healthcare by shifting the focus from simply reimbursing services to fix the broken ("fee-for-service"), to actually reimbursing for how medical providers produced health ("value-based care"). How do we actually improve the health of the patients we serve? Value-based care revolves around "population health" strategies, which aim to better manage "populations" of patients through improved, more proactive care design models.

Population health utilizes analytics to identify opportunities to improve health outcomes and assess the costs and benefits of clinical efforts designed to do so. Data in early population health efforts helped to illuminate an obvious truth that could no longer be ignored in these new models: *Healthy patients cost less than sick patients.*

In fee-for-service, this was an inconvenient truth that health systems chose to ignore, as they got paid a lot to fix sick patients. In population health models, it was foundational to strategy: If providers wanted to lower the costs they were now accountable for, they must improve health—with an evidenced-based, coordinated, and importantly, proactive approach. Manage diseases earlier and more effectively—or even better, prevent them in the first place.

By that time, I had seen the amount of human suffering—costly and preventable—which was tolerated in, or even facilitated by, fee-for-service models. It's one thing to read about health disparities among the poor; it's another thing to see them firsthand while being part of a larger healthcare system that fails to effectively address them.

So, while the 2010 IOM report supported the need for the population health model we were working on, reading it was still a gut-punch reality check for me at the time. It demonstrated on a national scale just how much our healthcare system profited from the brokenness of its own inefficiencies while ignoring and tolerating the suffering of the most vulnerable in our communities. It paralleled and magnified, through huge and grotesque numbers, the data we were seeing at our local level.

The report drew attention to the lack of sustainability of the cost curve of American healthcare and highlighted the areas where our costs were higher compared to other nations. A small percentage of those costs were related to medical fraud. Some were related to our disproportionately high administrative cost relative to other countries—which in a later 2018 analysis was calculated to be approximately four times higher in America than comparable countries, as a percentage of our overall healthcare spend at almost 9 percent.[4] But most was excess spent on futility—over-testing and over-treatment that did nothing to improve actual medical outcomes. The cost was calculated at $750 billion.[5] That number was paralyzing for me, Warren Buffett's economic tapeworm.

As we pursued new population health models at BHCHP, this report made any "significant" cost savings resulting from our efforts seem like futile drops in the bucket of a national system that didn't blink at irresponsibly wasting billions. As a clinician, and from an individual patient care level, this discrepancy didn't bother me or affect my clinical approaches with patients. But from a public health administrative perspective, I found it deflating. I struggled to get excited about saving a few million here or there, if in the bigger picture, any gain would almost instantly be canceled out by the inefficiencies of a profit-driven, fee-for-service system that could not care less.

The report wasn't necessarily a surprise to me, although the magnitude of waste was depressing. In the years prior to the study's release, I had increasingly become both fascinated and disheartened by the repeated patterns of waste in medicine routinely demonstrated in clinical trials. In my teaching rounds with residents or in our BHCHP medical provider meetings, I often would highlight articles and studies around the cost of medical futility.

Whether it was useless spinal fusions, unnecessary stents placed in blood vessels, hormone replacement therapies in both men and women that harmed rather than helped, or expensive diagnostic tests that had no clinical utility, so many studies were demonstrating our addiction to chasing reimbursements instead of science. Healthcare providers made hundreds of billions of dollars that we could not afford to waste as a nation on absolute futility. On the other end, they were withholding care from people who desperately needed it but could not afford it, even as these patients suffered and died expensively.

True, medicine was a vocation—especially at BHCP. Even more true, however, was that medicine was a massive industry that was focused, like all industries, on its financial success. Interventions, medications, and surgeries were often pushed more by industry and potential reimbursements than by scientific evidence.

The report mainly demonstrated the aggregate cost of all the waste in our medical system. The findings seemed egregious—because they were. The IOM report slapped me back into seeing a reality I was largely protected from while practicing in my public health bubble at BHCHP.

The report, however, also seemed incomplete.

BHCHP's Dr. Monica Bharel published an analysis of the cost of caring for 6,494 Medicaid patients in our program during 2010. The overall cost of our patients who suffered from homelessness was approximately 3.5 times higher than the average Medicaid patient. Of the total $149 million spent on this population, 10 percent of patients, or 649 people, were responsible for 48 percent of the cost. The average medical cost of those 649 patients in 2010 was $110,200.[6] For the most part, this cost wasn't related to the provision of unnecessary testosterone treatments or useless MRIs. Instead it was largely due to the late, complex, and desperate treatment of diseases that had progressed—neglected over years and lifetimes—to severe stages rather than being effectively managed or even prevented upstream at a fraction of the cost. Even in Boston, with all of its amazing resources for unhoused patients relative to other cities, we still saw a pattern of systemic neglect as diseases progressed, followed by expensive attempts to save the ship after it had already started to sink, despite all the clear warnings beforehand.

The IOM report had included and calculated the cost of futile tests, surgeries, and medications on one end of the healthcare access spectrum for those who could afford healthcare. However, it did not really capture the cost of these missed opportunities to prevent poor outcomes on the other.

As we were hemorrhaging money that was spiraling us down further into debt as a nation—a seemingly whopping $13 trillion at the time—it felt like there should be a much greater sense of urgency to address these inefficiencies. Instead, outside of BHCHP, all I saw was mainly collective shoulder shrugging.

How could we be so wasteful with unnecessary care for those who could afford it, while simultaneously being so expensively negligent and deficient in providing necessary care to sick patients who couldn't? One could dismiss it as all part of the free market setup of our healthcare system, but that seemed to be an expensive and inhumane dismissal—and horrifically inefficient, tolerating the hemorrhaging of taxpayer money and employer costs.

And those profiting the most from the waste were the ones who were being asked to fix it. Business models would never go against payment structures that dictated success, even if the intentions to do so were noble. It was a naïve and poor strategy to think otherwise.

Working with historically marginalized populations in this system within a public health model was a formula for burnout. I was constantly reminded of my grandfather's warning from over a decade earlier—*medicine is not a career; it is a vocation*—as I witnessed the consequences of the healthcare industry's obsession with profitability in those suffering around me.

In 2010, the same year that IOM released its report, the Affordable Care Act, or "Obamacare," was passed. Arguments and debates were just as contentious from both sides of the aisle as they had been in the 1990s. However, compared to the attempts to pass comprehensive healthcare reform 15 years earlier, politicians had perhaps learned enough political savvy after their past failures in navigating negotiations to keep a majority consensus.

There was also a growing bipartisan acceptance of the lack of sustainability of US medical costs. Just 40 years earlier, at the end of my grandfather's career in 1970, healthcare cost $75 billion, or only $356 annually per person—consuming 7.2 percent of our GDP. By the time the ACA passed in 2010, it was up to 18 percent of our GDP, costing $8,400 per person for an incredible $2.6 trillion per year. And it had grown by 150 percent since the last attempt at comprehensive healthcare reform legislation had failed under Clinton in 1994.[7]

Among its goals to increase access to care through Medicaid expansion, the ACA also included a more bipartisan idea to develop value-based care as the foundation of payment structures. Building on the ideas behind PCMH and other early "population health" models, the idea behind value-based care models was intuitive: Stop paying providers just to do things to patients (quantity). Instead, like almost all other industries, pay them based on how well they do their job of producing health in the populations they serve (quality). This made sense. In no other industry would somebody say, "I don't care about the results of your product. We will just keep paying you to produce more and more of it." It was no longer financially viable for our country to continue down this path.

Despite the contention around the ACA, subsequent legislation showed hints of support for this value-based focus from both sides of the aisle. A few years later in 2015, the Medicare Access and CHIP Reauthorization Act (MACRA) passed the House by a 392 to 97 vote, and was subsequently approved by the Senate with a 92 to 8 vote. This widely bipartisan supported bill fundamentally shaped how physicians would be paid and reimbursed by focusing on performance, quality, and value.[8]

However, to me, the IOM report revealed just how entrenched and metastatic our inefficiencies were in medicine. Even with the passing of the Affordable Care Act and its promises of improved access and payment design changes, the severity of our internal pathologies underlying American medicine didn't make me optimistic things would change any time soon.

―――

That same year, I experienced several patient losses that I struggled to shake off. In working with chronic homelessness, where the average life expectancy hovers around 50,[9] we must be able to stay functional while experiencing grief. As we deal with one loss, we must look up and keep working at the top of our game to prevent others as we constantly battle complicated social, medical, and behavioral health pathologies. This is, by far, my biggest challenge while working in our field. Over the course of their careers, medical providers learn how to professionally detach from severe grief to avoid paralysis at work. We seek condolence and motivation by telling ourselves "at least we made the suffering less" or "did the best we could under the circumstances."

However, over time, I—we, our BHCHP integrated care team—all became part of those "circumstances." We were dealing with a population suffering horrifically and dying young—often largely unassisted by a medical system that we told ourselves we were advocating to change, but which ultimately we were very much a part of.

We could see ourselves as advocates, yet at the end of the day, we were still part of the bigger system that failed our patients. In medicine, there's typically nobody more accountable for outcomes than primary care providers. Ultimately, those were *our* patients who were suffering and dying.

It became haunting to get to know good people, see their struggles, and feel powerless to help them as they transformed into ghosts before our eyes. Life was killing them. They were drowning, and the underlying forces driving their poor outcomes and death were confusing and often didn't seem impactable. Clinically, I felt lost—like I was always missing something.

As one of my medical students aptly described in frustration, as we were caring for a patient who suffered from chronic alcoholism and worsening liver cancer: "This feels like we are rearranging the deck chairs on the Titanic." The satisfaction from the wins at that time were increasingly negated by the pain of the defeats.

The most frustrating part was knowing I was practicing at a healthcare organization with more resources, financial support, and leadership than any in the nation. And yet, there I was feeling like I was burning out, seemingly unable to have the same strength, resilience, and perseverance as the other BHCHP providers. And it wasn't that they were callused or aloof. They cared more than anybody. Deeply. They showed sustained strength and determined altruism—at incredible levels. I felt inspired to witness it, but deflated when I couldn't replicate it.

I absolutely loved my job and the people I worked with. Yet each patient loss was getting harder. I couldn't really envision being able to continue this for many years longer.

This all made the decision to leave versus stay feel excruciating, as my wife and I were trying to figure out what was best for our young family. We had no family in Boston. Being raised in Los Angeles, I found the cold weather intolerable; I never toughened up. Every September around Labor Day, the tree in our front yard in the Boston suburb of Needham would obnoxiously start to drop leaves, way ahead of autumn protocols I was used to elsewhere. In the winter of 2010 to 2011, when we were debating our major life decisions, we had over 80 inches of snow. There was one patch on my driveway that I inevitably, even when I knew it was there, would slip on while shoveling—every time.

Even more challenging was being in Boston, after growing up a Lakers fan in Los Angeles during the 1980s when our dynamic "Showtime" Lakers were frequently matched in the finals against the cantankerous Boston Celtics. In 2009, when the Lakers lost to the Celtics in the NBA finals, the obnoxiousness that radiated out from my neighbors in Boston was brutal. In 2011, when we came back to beat the Celtics in the finals, the revenge was awesome.

Between the Celtics, the cost of living, and the weather, I struggled to justify if loving the job to the extent I did was enough to stay. With my commitment to National Health Corp already completed the year before, my kids about to enter grade school, and our desire to provide stability for our family without moving all the time heightened, it felt like the option was to leave then or stay for the long term.

In February of that year, we were late getting my five-year old son out the door to attend a birthday party.

"Dad, we've got to get in the ca-h!" he yelled in exasperation.

He'd dropped his hard R. That was it. Visions of him 20 years in the future in a Celtic's jersey watching a game in the "Gah-den" and yelling and screaming R-less profanities and insults was enough to push us over the edge.

We made the tough call to move, leaving behind an incredible job, patients I loved, and an eclectic group of amazing neighbors who had become family in our small, double cul-de-sac Needham neighborhood.

While deciding to leave Boston was hard, deciding on where to move to was even harder. After struggling to decide between some really cool options that were ultimately narrowed down to Denver and Raleigh, a literal coin flip broke through our indecision on June 30, 2010, on a small grassy hill outside of Boston Medical Center.

Heads.

Heads meant Raleigh. The decision was made. I was going to

work at WakeMed, the main hospital system serving North Carolina's Wake County.

Leaving was more difficult than I'd expected. I could and did reference cost of living, lack of family, horrifically cold weather, the annoying 17-ringed Boston Celtics, or a fear of my children developing a Boston accent as reasons for leaving. But despite all my anguish with the decision, in reality, burnout and frustration made the decision to leave Boston for me, even if I hadn't realized it—or wanted to admit to it. I felt like I was giving up. Deep down, I couldn't help but feel like I was abandoning my patients.

The hardest part of leaving was saying goodbye to the patients I'd grown close to. Our other collaborative team members helped to ensure there would be continuity of care when I left. But it still felt like abandonment. Saying goodbye to one patient proved particularly hard.

9
ALONE

Peter had a reputation for being difficult, with a quick temper that often crossed over to violence on the streets, resulting in frequent associated injuries and incarcerations. He was confrontational and often explosive during his bad times. He was brilliant and often very friendly during his good times.

After enjoying early success in his career in his 20s, a series of personal tragedies and associated losses tore Peter's life apart. The most traumatic involved witnessing the sudden and violent loss of his young wife in an accident. The mental health crash that followed resulted in him losing his job and most of his family and social connections.

The pain of this dramatic 180 in his life—the realization of the potential that was lost—tormented him. It served as a reminder of how quickly life can turn for any of us.

"It was great, and then it was essentially over ... just like that," he recalled.

He was surprised and disappointed by his self-perceived lack of resilience. And he was impacted by how others saw him when he was homeless.

"The most painful thing is how people treat you," he lamented.

"Nobody treats you like a normal person. Some will treat you with pity, most with disdain, but nobody treats you like a normal person." This observation mentally tortured him. He had several unsuccessful suicide attempts when he felt he couldn't take it anymore.

Peter would be the first to admit that he was not very endearing. It took some time to develop our relationship. By the time I started to care for him when he was in his late 40s, his decades of chronic homelessness had taken their toll, leaving him with amputated digits from frostbite, head trauma from fights, and end-stage liver disease from heavy alcohol use. None of these hardships and episodes were enough to shock him back onto a different, healthier path.

His struggle with alcoholism started after the death of his wife. He hit it hard early and never really took his foot off the gas—with no periods of sobriety or enrollment in treatment programs.

As his liver disease got worse, he inevitably spent more time in our respite care facility, as he was often too sick to be on the streets. It was during these stays that I had opportunities to develop a trusting clinical relationship with him, where I could get to know him away from the chaos of the streets. This ultimately resulted in facilitating close follow-up with me as an outpatient, when he was not in respite.

We did see some intermittent improvement in his outcomes over the years. Progress wasn't easy. In fact, it was painful every step of the way. One step forward could easily be negated with two steps back in the context of an intoxicated interaction or eruption in the clinic.

One such eruption happened just a few weeks before I left Boston. By that time, his liver disease had progressed to the point where his MELD score, a risk stratification tool that looks at different clinical factors to predict mortality, was over 30. This meant his chance of death in the next three months was over 50 percent. He was turning into a ghost, and he and I knew it.

He came into the clinic intoxicated. He was triggered—angry about everything and anything, but when it came down to it, nothing he could specifically articulate. As he was yelling, he developed a nosebleed—not uncommon in people with advanced liver disease due to low platelet counts and deficient clotting factors. As the blood continued to drip from his nose throughout my clinic, he became increasingly incensed that I would not prescribe him Percocet for his pain.

Peter's addiction had always been primarily to alcohol, but occasionally when he was desperate, he would replace it with Percocet/narcotics. He knew my policy around narcotic pain medications (almost always more harm than good, especially in the context of non-specific pain as he was describing, and his associated addiction history). But when intoxicated and desperate, he'd occasionally still take a shot. This was one of those days.

My persistent refusal, while predictable, wasn't sitting well with him. As he raged across my clinic, bleeding everywhere and tossing my papers as a sign of frustration (but I don't think intimidation), he appeared weaker and more jaundiced than ever. He left a mess behind him as he stormed out.

Two days later, sober, he returned to the clinic. In his moments of sobriety, he was one of the more articulate and intelligent people I had ever met. Occasionally during those interactions, he would provide incredible insights—into homelessness, or life in general.

This time, he was particularly introspective—perhaps feeling a need to address the conflict of the bloody-nose interaction from a few days before.

He wasn't apologetic, but I think in his own way, he was trying to explain his actions. I was taken aback by how he started the conversation.

"Do you know what my biggest fear in life is?"

Not waiting for me to respond, he quickly answered his own question: "Dying a bum."

He recognized what was happening with his health. His recent deterioration seemed to be snowballing in the past few months, with more respite care admissions related to his worsening liver disease. He had been tracking his MELD score and its associated "clock." Time was running out, and he knew it.

Peter was coming to grips with his inevitable mortality. He wasn't going to be able to flip the script, dramatically changing the storyline in the last chapter of his life into a surprising, happy ending. He'd never really displayed a real interest in doing so. He'd been resigned to his fate.

"A bum?" I asked.

"Alone."

Loneliness is one of the greatest pains of homelessness. As patients start coming to grips with advanced disease and the dying process, they're reminded of the path that led them to their current reality.

In the fiction of books and movies, we're accustomed to the last-minute, dramatic pivot to a happy ending. Everything turns out well. We're relieved and happy.

There's often a type of survival mechanism of hope in our patients that helps them dream that theirs could be the case that gets turned around. They long to feel hope for better days. For relief. Maybe even for a cure. Deep down, it's what keeps many people going—desperately clinging to hope that it will end differently because it simply *cannot* end like this.

The reality is, however, that it often does. It just ends.

No family members rushing back in to love and support them at the end. No long-lost friends reconnecting. Just sickness and illness and loneliness, synergizing and snowballing to ensure one last dehumanizing insult as they leave this world alone. Bodies found on the streets. In hotel rooms. In encampment sites. Or in lonely hospital beds without visitors. To die alone seems to be the ultimate final insult of the dehumanization of homelessness. Perhaps this is why it was Peter's greatest fear.

Three weeks later, I saw Peter on my last day of clinic at Boston Health Care for the Homeless. I had intentionally scheduled him for my final day and reminded him about this date a few times. However, in the context of intermittent intoxication and the confusion that comes with the "encephalopathy" of advanced liver disease, he hadn't remembered. He knew I was leaving, but he was surprised this was my last day. We discussed his case, his symptoms, and the transitional plans that included him following up with an excellent clinician he knew from respite.

At the end of our visit, he thanked me for everything, I talked about what an honor it was to be part of his care, and he went his way. Our parting went well, but admittedly seemed a bit forced and "not enough" given our history, what we had worked through together, and where he was in life. He referenced a bus he had to catch. I had a lot more patients on the schedule and was already 30 minutes behind. The day continued on.

A few hours later, a "code blue" call came from the lobby. Per protocol, everybody rushed down as quickly as we could to help. We were always prepared to deal with the worst, but typically code blues were called by staff erring on the side of caution. A seizure, fainting, shortness of breath—only rarely were they life-threatening.

This time I rushed down to see Peter in the lobby, sitting in a chair, surrounded by nurses who always seemed to somehow beat most of the medical providers to these codes. (Even when I tried to sprint and fly downstairs, it seemed I could never get there first. I'm convinced they had some maze of secret nurse-passages.)

Peter was sweating profusely and somewhat short of breath. He was drenched, and appeared as jaundiced and emaciated as ever.

In non-urgent situations, the primary care provider who knew the patient would typically take over. So I went over to Peter and asked what happened.

"I think I overdid it," he replied.

He explained: After our visit earlier in the morning, he had taken the bus back to his new transitional housing unit, which he had moved into a few months earlier. It was the first time he had been housed for years. Concerned he would miss me if he waited for the later bus, he decided to walk back to the clinic, about two miles, in abnormally hot and humid weather for Boston. With his liver disease, it was too much for him.

After a few minutes and a few glasses of water, he felt better—annoyed by all the commotion, but better.

"I wanted to give you this—for your boys."

He opened his hand to reveal a small teddy bear key chain. The bear had a big heart in the middle that read, "I love Boston." It was scratched and didn't appear to be new.

He looked up, embarrassed.

"It's not much, but I want them to have something to remember Boston by."

For the second time in the past few weeks, tears formed in his eyes. He quickly got up to leave, begrudgingly accepting my attempts at gratitude while ignoring, stubbornly per usual, my pleas to continue to rest, especially as a thunderstorm was starting outside, breaking through the thick summer humidity he had just walked through.

"I'll be alright," he insisted. He clearly wanted to get out of there.

He would take the bus back. A staff member tried to walk him back to the bus stop to ensure he would be OK, but after Peter told him to screw off, we ended up just watching from the window to make sure he made it through the pouring rain and driving winds to get safely on the bus.

That would be the last day either Peter or I would be in that clinic. The following week, Peter missed his clinic appointment with his new provider. A month later, during my new employee orientation at WakeMed, I would get a text that Peter had passed away. He had died in the middle of the night in a local Boston hospital ICU bed.

Alone.

10

SCATTERED SAFETY NETS

North Carolina was one of the states that didn't initially expand Medicaid under the ACA. When I arrived in Raleigh, I quickly learned how much this limited the health-related resources relative to my experience in Boston.

In many of the lower-income neighborhoods surrounding WakeMed, many people lacked medical insurance. In fact, WakeMed itself was in the census tract with historically the highest rate of uninsured residents, hovering around one-third of the population. What Medicaid had provided in terms of social and medical safety nets in Massachusetts, the community had to collaborate to piece together in Raleigh. Out of this necessity arose a fascinating collection of safety net clinics, social service systems, and faith-based organizations that worked to fill in the gaps.

From a medical perspective, these efforts were led by free charity clinics, federally qualified centers, and some local neighborhood doctors who had served Raleigh's lowest-income neighborhoods for years. These medical providers made sacrifices in their own careers, and paychecks, to serve the patients nobody else would. These providers desperately tried, the best they could, to manage the health of patients who had very little resources.

When I moved to Raleigh, I intentionally selected a job at the main safety net hospital in Wake County. As I got settled in the area, I struggled to identify the people providing homeless healthcare locally—until I discovered that Joanne (big surprise!) had a connection, Brooks Ann McKinney. I vividly remember Joanne describing her in one word, "firecracker," then further explaining "she does not mess around."

She was right. Brooks Ann, with her master's in social work, had been serving those suffering from homelessness for years, including developing respite care models that eventually led to her serving on the National Respite Care Provider's Network. There, she became friends with Joanne, who also served on the council. Brooks Ann's passion pushed her to innovate, implement, learn from, and continuously evolve models of care, especially around homeless outreach and respite care models. Joanne got me in touch with Brooks Ann, who subsequently directed me to Dr. Jim Hartye.

When I left Boston Health Care for the Homeless, we had more than 330 staff members serving our patients. In Raleigh, it was just Dr. Hartye, Brooks Ann, and a handful of other clinicians—including a homeless outreach nurse, Jane Smith, who I would later work with on our team at WakeMed. Granted, the homeless population in Raleigh was approximately 10 percent that of Boston. But still, it was an incredibly small skeleton staff that was trying to meet the healthcare needs of the local homeless population.

Dr. Hartye worked as both a physician at WakeMed and a provider at the local federally funded healthcare for the homeless clinic. At the latter, he was on a clinical island. He spent his days treating the overwhelming pathologies of the homeless population the best he could.

Soon after I arrived in Raleigh, Dr. Hartye allowed me to shadow him at his clinic. It was small and crowded—every inch utilized out of necessity. The contrast of his daily clinical routine to what I experienced in Boston was stark. His interactions were less social and less relaxed. There wasn't as much laughing. In an over-scheduled, under-staffed clinic, he didn't have much time for small talk. He efficiently pushed through each day with a quiet determination to keep his head above water, so he could help as many patients as possible do the same. He didn't have the luxury of going too far down paths of chronic disease management or preventive health, instead needing to spend his time putting out fires and stopping hemorrhaging.

However, no matter how busy he was, Dr. Hartye showed an innate ability to make people feel important and listened to. His compassion was immediately evident in his interactions, which were genuine and not forced.

He also didn't have the luxury of an integrated care team. He didn't have somebody like Dr. McGahee working in the room next to him, as I'd had in Boston. He was a primary care provider and psychiatrist all in one.

Fortunately for him, his years of experience had made him truly a mental health expert. Most of the 13 patients we saw that morning in that three-and-a-half hour session suffered primarily from mental health issues.

His incredible patience inside the clinic was contrasted by his aggressive advocacy outside of it. Neither he nor Brooks Ann were hesitant to shine a bright light on the inefficiencies of the systems they saw failing their patients on a daily basis.

Their work was inspirational.

It was also exhausting. Out of necessity, they had developed a classic "hero model," wherein a small number of uniquely altruistic healthcare providers were willing to make personal sacrifices to help those patients who everybody else was ignoring. They accepted less pay while working longer and harder hours as they cared for challenging patients nobody else wanted—all with an amazing sense of purpose and mission.

Hero models are inspirational. They show us what's possible while providing incredible role models. They display a contrast between what currently exists and what might actually be possible through innovation, dedication, and hard work.

The danger of these models, however, is that reproducing them is nearly impossible. And typically, burnout is almost inevitable. Hero models pretend the impossible is possible. They're exactly what Jim O'Connell worked to guard against as he developed BHCHP over the years.

Large-scale transformation can't depend on the hero model. It's not sustainable. We can't strategize around individuals making extreme financial and quality-of-life sacrifices as the foundation for sustainable, widely-implemented public health models. We need payment reform to support the good work being done, not sporadic inspirational providers who make personal sacrifices to work in its gaps.

Additionally, an otherwise disinterested community can point to these hero models as evidence that "at least something is being done," thereby providing a cover for a continued lack of more comprehensive action. Systems are often looking more for cover than inspiration—a box checked so they don't have to make larger, more significant changes. This assuaged guilt can impede the sense of urgency to address difficult but obvious problems.

Dr. Hartye and Brooks Ann fiercely pushed back against these tendencies up until the day they left Raleigh.

Dr. Hartye would move to Kentucky a few months after I arrived in Raleigh, leaving a huge, leaderless void in our local homeless health programs. Brooks Ann wasn't too far behind, as she headed out west to the mountains of Asheville.

11

THE DICHOTOMY

I began my work with WakeMed in their downtown Raleigh primary care clinic in September of 2011. This part of the city was going through a significant development stage at the time. In the decade that followed, as the population in Wake County continued to explode, empty lots would turn into high-end apartment complexes and office buildings. The city was growing and thriving with new bars, trendy restaurants, and summer street festivals.

The clinic itself was in the middle of it all. It had just opened a few months before my arrival. A converted spa, it had a unique layout with a waterfall feature in its lobby and an old sauna in the patient bathroom. The clinic resided on the first floor of a large office building and shared a wall with the popular and trendy Sosta Café. Our close proximity next door often allowed our clinic to smell like his freshly baked brownies in the mornings. I quickly developed an ordering system of banging on our shared wall to expedite my order.

For years, we were the only primary care clinic in downtown Raleigh.

As my panel developed, it evolved into a fascinating mix of

patients. One on end, we saw patients from the local businesses, universities, and political offices, as we were only about a half-mile from the state capital. These patients would take advantage of the growing trend of establishing a doctor near work, to minimize time off and increase access to care. On the other end, we were also just a few blocks east of the lowest income neighborhoods in Raleigh—ones where life expectancies were more than 12 years lower compared to the wealthier northwestern suburbs. Not surprisingly, we started to see growing volumes of patients who suffered from homelessness and increasingly lacked other medical options walking into our clinic for care.

The clinic was increasingly capturing some of the most complex and highest-risk patients in our community while simultaneously engaging many of the area's corporate and government leaders. This setup provided a unique perspective around the health of—and on a larger scale, societal dichotomy between—the rich and poor. Their human physiologies were similar. Their social drivers of health were starkly different.

One day in the fall of 2012, just a year after I started at Wake-Med, I heard an already very recognizable loud voice coming from our waiting room, sounding a bit louder and more intoxicated than usual. I walked out, past the bathroom sauna and hallway waterfall, into the lobby to find Craig. He was engaging in a primarily one-sided, boisterous conversation with a local corporate CEO sitting on his left and a state politician on his right.

It was a sight.

Craig was moderately obese, in his mid-40s, with a long, grey, disheveled beard. He had arrived 45 minutes early for his appointment, both to get out of the rain but also to charge his phone. Per usual, he had brought all his bags to clinic with him—about four or five suitcases. His phone was plugged in through an abnormally long, neon-green charging cord.

He was wearing a grungy pair of, unfortunately, urine-soaked pants and a T-shirt with large middle finger artwork in the middle that nicely complemented the inappropriate message he had tattooed across his knuckles.

Craig was an engaging conversationalist—partly because he was so genuinely excited to talk to anybody. He had a manic way of moving his hands and raising his voice when he spoke, but it was more engaging than intimidating. His speech was pressured, yet his tangential runs were routinely punctuated by pauses to ask questions. This made the conversation feel more two-way than the typical manic, pressured speech of patients who suffered from bipolar disease.

Neither the local politician nor the CEO appeared frustrated. Both actually seemed fascinated as Craig continued to talk and editorialize on something that had apparently been on the TV in our waiting room a few minutes earlier. In fact, the CEO was already done with his visit and was just hanging out, having seemingly been drawn into the conversation as he was leaving the clinic.

I stood there waiting and actually got wrapped up in listening to Craig before any of them noticed I was there. I brought back the politician first for his appointment, leaving the CEO and Craig to continue their discussions.

Both Craig and the politician had diabetes.

The politician was doing excellent. He was working with a trainer, starting a diet with his supportive wife, and beginning to routinely use the treadmill in his basement each morning before work. Twelve minutes later, we were walking out of the office, giving each other clinical high-fives, as he was meeting all the diabetic goals that would determine not only his long-term health outcomes but also the clinical quality measures I was being held accountable for in primary care. He had done all the work and tapped into the great resources available to him. I was going to clinically get credit for his success.

Craig was next. He said his goodbye to the CEO (still there), gathered all his bags, and walked down the long hallway, past the waterfall, to the exam room. Thirty minutes later, I was still just trying to go through his confusing bag of pill bottles, expired insulin syringes mixed in with food, and a collection of spilled vitamins and medications at the bottom of the bag—all as he was editorializing and monologuing on some topic concerning the Milli Vanilli lip-synching controversy.

Craig's A1C, which is a measure of diabetic control, had improved from 14.1 to 10.6 after he stopped his habit of drinking six to eight Mountain Dews a day. He admitted it was tough, but he was able to do it. While the politician had just nailed a 6.4 A1C the visit before, I was much more excited over Craig's results. I knew this represented an improvement that moved him back from the "edge of the cliff" of possible hospitalizations and poor outcomes due to high sugars and associated acidosis, to just "really poor control." This meant if we could continue the progress, we could keep him out of the hospital—which was awesome, as he didn't do well when he was admitted. While I recognized he would still be a ding on my diabetic quality measures where the A1C goal was set at below 8, I was pleasantly shocked we were able to get it down to these levels in the context of his social barriers and associated lack of access to healthy foods, exercise, and insulin. I would get credit for being an effective provider for the politician, even though his diet, trainer, and wife really got him to the goal. So it balanced out—unwarranted credit on one end, and unwarranted blame on the other.

I billed the same codes for both Craig and the politician. We would get reimbursed more for the politician's visit given his insurance plan, although Craig's appointment took four times longer and would make my clinical performance appear worse.

We were never able to convince Craig to see a mental health provider, or really engage with any issue besides his diabetes. He refused vaccines. He had zero interest in smoking cessation. He had a strong conspiracy theory against cholesterol medications. But he did allow us to manage his blood sugars.

A few months later, Craig suddenly stopped coming into the clinic. We discovered he was arrested and incarcerated for grand larceny. He would end up dying in prison a few years later.

The CEO and politician are still doing well.

12

COMFORTABLY BROKEN

Change management is an essential part of any industry. It involves helping people in an organization or company understand, accept, and engage with changes necessary to improve and evolve. This engagement is critical.

Even when something is as broken as our American healthcare system, and the need for change is intuitive, change can still be resisted. The familiar may be broken, but it's still familiar and, therefore, comfortable. This is especially true when the familiar, comfortable, and broken have been profitable.

A reflexive "no" coupled with excuses is much easier than a "yes" requiring innovative solutions. In the face of a potential change, those reflexively and often loudly dishing out the objections and "can't be dones" can then naturally assume the somewhat narcissistic but comfortable contrarian role. In this role, one doesn't need to think, try, or expend any energy. They can simply sit back and criticize those trying to implement the necessary change. Even though they're doing nothing, they get to sound intellectually superior through their criticism—as they *must* know something that those pushing for change don't know in their ignorant naivety and advocacy.

Medicine, as with any large, complicated, and profitable industry, is filled with such contrarians. Up front, they loudly voice why and how a necessary change won't work. And then, they resist that change in order to turn their predictions of failure into reality, securing the rights to an "I told you so" validation. You can find these contrarians at the forefront of any change initiative. Relatively speaking, they're often a small minority—but they're also typically pretty loud. They can present major barriers to the cultural changes needed for progress, kill morale, and be particularly harmful when the necessary change is as significant as it is in medicine.

Importantly, they must not be confused with those who are truly engaged, giving constructive feedback and criticism to better evolve the change. These are your best advocates.

This differentiation is typically easily made, as motive is usually transparent.

I felt myself going down that stubborn, contrarian path in 2013—not yet too loud, but reflexively pessimistic about any clinical initiative proposed by others sticking their necks out to advocate for change. My four years in Boston included constant change and innovation. I found it exciting and interesting, but it always seemed like we should be doing more—that we must be chasing the wrong things, as nothing seemed to truly "flip the switch" to the necessary extent. Patients continued to suffer expensively and die young in the context of homelessness, amidst a culture where larger medical systems tolerated poor outcomes. These systems didn't seem to share a sense of urgency, or really even an interest to do better, despite public vows and statements.

I hated knowing I was part of the "system." I didn't want to be part of the hypocrisy or its failures. And change requires patience, skill, and courage to continue working inside chaos and brokenness, while still affecting outcomes. Complaining about what I resented was much easier than trying to fix it. If I wasn't part of any change initiative, I could at least internally point my finger at everybody else when things failed—and they often did. I didn't want the fingers—especially my own—pointed at me. I didn't want to be set up for failure and the associated guilt.

The failures in our field of medicine are pretty brutal. In public health, they often involve deadly, expensive, and devastating outcomes. I felt myself increasingly becoming one of medicine's reflexive contrarians. It bothered me that that I was letting this happen so early in my career.

―――

It was at this time, in 2013, that I was approached to become the chief medical officer of a new accountable care organization (ACO) at WakeMed.

ACOs were formed as a foundational aspect of the Affordable Care Act—a key strategy component around value-based payment models. The overall idea was that groups of medical providers would work together to manage their population of patients and be held accountable for how they accomplished the "triple aim" of value-based care—patient outcomes, patient satisfaction, and overall medical cost. These three components, collectively, provided a balance that prevented the pushing of any one component too hard. Medical providers would be held accountable for, and increasingly reimbursed based on, how much it cost to effectively manage the health of their population of patients—on how they actually produced health, not simply on how many services they provided.

WakeMed, as an independent community hospital, partnered to form our ACO with a group of more than 350 independent, local primary care providers—providers who were self-employed and had, to date, resisted (or really, survived outside of) the trend of going to work for large hospital systems.

When my grandfather practiced medicine, almost all physicians were self-employed. With increased regulations, complicated payer demands, and less certain business models, that number shrunk over time. By the time the ACA passed in 2011, the percentage of self-employed physicians was down to around 52 percent; by 2020, it dropped to 44 percent.[1]

From a community perspective, there's a benefit to having primary care physicians remain independent. They can answer to their patients without necessarily being influenced by the larger goals of healthcare systems.

The ACO allowed us to partner with these independent physicians to develop clinical strategies and resources to help improve the health outcomes of hundreds of thousands of patients in our community.

The ACO also held some potential and promises to address some very fundamental flaws of our healthcare system through payment reform ... maybe. Primary care had been burned before by promises of payment reforms that would better reimburse and reward for their relative contributions to patients' health. However, there was still reason for optimism that this time may be different.

I was intrigued by the position and larger concept. The model could help address some of the most significant pathologies underlying medicine's historic and costly inefficiencies. *Healthy patients cost less than sick patients—and are more satisfied. Maximize health instead of expensively fixing the broken.*

Running this model with a group of independent primary care providers, especially ones who had excelled in implementing the patient-centered medical home model in the preceding years, was too good to pass up—even in the context of my early-career Grumpledump transformation.

Given my experience with PCMH and "population health" with what was considered a high-risk homeless population, and likely in the context of my general geekiness, I was approached by leadership about the ACO's chief medical officer (CMO) position. My growing curmudgeonness was still disguised. Deep down, I was excited about the model's potential, both clinically and as a way to drag me out of my worsening pessimism. *Perhaps it could make me accountable to help fix our problems in medicine instead of just complaining about them.*

Still, I procrastinated with my decision ... up until the application deadline on December 30, 2013, when I finally submitted it a few hours before midnight. At least I did not have to flip a coin this time.

I spent the next seven years working to navigate our ACO and its 400-plus primary care providers through the chaotic but exciting beginnings of value-based care. Initially, I spent half of my time as CMO of the ACO while maintaining the other half seeing patients in my downtown Raleigh clinic. We were one of the largest ACOs in the county. Our strategy was relatively straightforward and therefore really fun, given the strength of our primary care providers. Our success as an ACO, and in our associated measures, was simply the sum of the success of our providers in their individual patient interactions.

We got buy-in from our providers early on. They realized the change away from fee-for-service to value-based care was inevitable. It was going to happen with or without us, so we decided we may as well take the lead. We then provided them with the tools and resources needed to be successful. We flipped historically antagonistic relationships between healthcare providers and healthcare insurance companies into productive collaborations.

Our ACOs saw excellent outcomes. This was almost an inevitability, considering we were combining our strong, community-based primary care base with a safety net hospital partner—with its roots also based in the community—and a progressive leadership who saw the potential of the model to improve patient care.

It was awesome ... and it was also somewhat boring.

I became distracted after only my first year.

13

HOTSPOTTING

When ACOs like ours started, they quickly became focused on one glaring statistic: 1 percent of patients were responsible for a significant portion, typically 25 percent, of the total cost we were being held accountable for. For perspective, as a nation we spend more on the healthcare of 1 percent of Americans than we do on our military[1] or on K–12 public education.[2] This *1 percent of patients equals approximately 25 percent of cost* stat held true at all levels—national, local, clinic, and even down to the individual healthcare provider level when we looked at it in our ACO.

An entire "population health" IT industry was developed around this statistic. The market became flooded with companies selling their ability to create proprietary predictive analytics that could and would identify who these "1 percent" patients *would* be in the future (not the ones who were already historically costly). A ton of data points could be captured and used to guide who we should invest our time and resources in to help avoid future high costs and poor outcomes.

It was an intuitive strategy to start early population health efforts with this 1 percent. A patient population of 300,000 seemed overwhelming to begin transformation efforts with. But what about 3,000? That seemed much more manageable. For a provider with a panel of 3,000 or so patients, starting with their "top 30" felt very doable. It was a great place to start.

As ACOs started to implement their strategies, working to identify and then engage these patients, a second stat could no longer be ignored: The vast majority of health outcomes, an estimated 80 percent, and their associated costs have absolutely *nothing* to do with what happens in our hospitals and medical clinics. Even though that's where we spend 90 percent of our over $4 trillion in medical costs—on direct medical care—the reality is that it doesn't influence outcomes much.[3] This one statistic might sum up our historical flaws in American healthcare better than any other. It was a statistic we could ignore in fee-for-service models where providers got paid well to fix (or at least try to fix) that which broke in the community.

However, the stat became impossible to ignore in models where we got paid for how we actually produced *health*. If we were going to be successful in such models, we would need to move outside the walls of our comfortable, historically well-compensated medical silos and into the much-more-difficult-to-control community. Most health systems had zero idea how to actually do this, flying blind as they started in their attempts.

As an ACO, we would meet monthly with insurance companies and review their high utilizing patients who we cared for. Typically, these patients would accumulate high costs due to multiple hospitalizations or ER visits. Three or four hospitalizations, or 12 or 13 ER visits, in a year were the norm for these high utilizers. However, the contrast between the healthcare utilization of these commercially insured ACO patients and the chronically homeless patients I had historically served was stark: Those experiencing homelessness would often have this level of ER and hospital utilization over a few weeks.

The early payment models of value-based care involved shared savings. In most arrangements, we would keep up to half of the savings our care provided against expected cost, depending on how well we did with quality measures. The insurance companies would keep the other half. The future state of reimbursement we were moving toward was "full risk"—wherein providers would keep all the savings if present, but on the flip side, they would eat the cost if the group of patients spent above established targets. So, for example, if a group of 1,000 Insurance X patients were calculated to have an expected cost during the year of $1,000,000, and they ended up costing only $800,000, the ACO and its providers would keep all of the $200,000. If they ended up costing $1,200,000, then the ACO (and its providers) would pay Insurance X $200,000. As an ACO, we constantly talked about preparing for these potential future "at risk" models, often with trepidation.

But what about populations wherein we were *already* at risk?

As I mentioned, North Carolina was one of the states that didn't initially expand Medicaid through the ACA—nor would it until the end of 2023. Wake County still had tens of thousands of people without healthcare insurance.

Our hospital's administration was now more familiar with the concepts of value-based care and speaking its vernacular. Through our work with the ACO, they appreciated the importance of better managing this "top 1 percent." We were able to approach the financial leadership of the hospital about an intuitive idea that had previously fallen on deaf ears just less than two years earlier: The same thing we were presently doing for Medicare and the commercially insured patients in our ACO, we should do internally for the uninsured patients the hospital served—controlling cost by better managing our most vulnerable and highest-cost patients.

We came prepared with data from an analysis of the uninsured care our hospital had provided for the community. As expected, 27 percent of the cost of caring for the tens of thousands of uninsured residents we saw each year was attributed to 1 percent of the patients. The cost was tens of millions of dollars, the vast majority of which we never recovered. We were, essentially, already "at full risk" for these very complex patients. When there was no insurance company—no payer—*we* were the payer.

Hospitals across America had tolerated this brokenness for years, taking huge financial losses on those uninsured patients in their communities who had no resources to improve their health. Hospitals made enough on their insured patients to compensate, and many of the financial losses could be adjusted for through provisions of government payment adjustments and tax write-offs. But while historically there was always enough money to go around to absorb these losses, tolerating avoidable human suffering is always a bad strategy—yes, morally, but also financially. The argument was easy and intuitive: If we are already basically "at risk" financially, let's act like it.

Our arguments revolved around both financial benefits as well as the ethical implications. Our mission was "to serve with outstanding and compassionate care to all." In our new population health mindset, this required us to be more proactive in addressing the expensive suffering of patients who were routinely collapsing into our safety net ERs and inpatient beds. We would need to do a better job of getting into the community.

Our uniquely mission-focused hospital leadership not only bought into but wholly supported our early visions, efforts, and innovations around how we managed our sickest and most vulnerable patients—and they have continued to do so ever since.

In late 2014, separate from our ACO efforts, our hospital started a relatively basic *hotspotter* model for our local uninsured patients, without support or resources from insurance companies.

The model was based on an approach described by Atul Gawande three years earlier in a 2011 *New Yorker* article about Dr. Jeffery Brenner in Camden, New Jersey. The approach involved using data to identify high-utilizing patients and provide intensive team-based case management to help link them with outpatient care and social services.[4] When I first read the article while still in Boston, I found the model fascinating. It had the potential to make medicine both more humane and more efficient.

I was partnered with Jennifer McLucas, a licensed therapist who had supervised our behavioral health teams at WakeMed, to help build and develop the team. For the next several years, I would help run this hotspotter model while simultaneously continuing my work as chief medical officer of our ACO (and continuing to see patients in my downtown clinic). This resulted in crazy hours, but it also provided a unique opportunity to participate in the early evolution of value-based care from multiple different perspectives.

As we started the hotspotter model, we were approached by various population health tech companies wanting to sell us their analytics to help identify the sickest patients we should engage. We were surprised to discover that, at the time, many of their secret, proprietary, expensive algorithms excluded people experiencing homelessness or severe mental health issues. Based on the historical fee-for models from which they collected their data, these conditions were found to be "not impactable." This wasn't because they *actually* weren't impactable, but more because the analytics could only feed and be built from our previous experiences and outcomes in fee-for-service approaches where we had no idea what we were doing in managing severe social or mental health pathologies, nor did we really care.

These new tech companies rushing to the market had nothing to draw their data from besides the historically broken. For example, traditional case management programs typically involved simple telephonic outreach to engage patients; after three unsuccessful attempts, patients who did not answer would be placed in the "didn't answer, not impactable" category. But it's hard to answer a phone if you don't have one, or if you are working two different jobs to make ends meet without the luxury of waiting around all day to talk to an insurance company case manager.

These analytic models had a long way to go, especially when used in high-risk models that attempted to identify "the top 1 percent." We didn't want to pay a lot of money to be experimental guinea pigs, so we developed our own analytics through the data in our electronic medical record (EMR), EPIC. It got us 95 percent of the way there; we didn't need advanced analytics to identify that the person who came into our ER 10 times last week was probably worth taking a look at.

When we turned the data analysis on, what we found was disturbing—and familiar.

Analytics are critical to population health. They allow us to identify our flaws, expose them, and continue to expose them repeatedly until we can no longer ignore them.

The data fed through our EMR was real-time—unlike with the ACO, where we would capture data sent to us from the insurance companies and Medicare on a three-month "claims delay." This real-time EMR data allowed us to view the cost and suffering as they were happening, not afterward.

We developed different columns to fully capture our different types of risks. First, we had an overall risk score, which we built around an equation that factored utilization, medical conditions, behavioral health conditions, and social determinants into the equations. A second column separated out and highlighted just the utilization piece of the overall risk score. It would give any ER visit over the preceding three months one point and any hospitalization three points. A third column reflected the total utilization *across the community*, capturing data from our two other local healthcare systems through a data feed, as they also used EPIC for their electronic medical record system. Finally, we had a column that displayed total utilization just in the past two weeks—a true "hotspotter" column. A patient with no historical utilization who suddenly was in the ER eight to nine times in the past two weeks was someone we should be running toward before it was too late—before the suffering snowballed into bad outcomes or, even worse, death. Too often with the ACO, these are the patients we would be discussing around the table *after* they had already died or accumulated hundreds of thousands of dollars in costs, before the three-month claims-delayed data would flag them.

This two-week report added a sense of urgency—and opportunity—to our efforts. It changed the conversations from the retrospective "oh, that's stinks; the damage is done" with claims-delayed data to a more active clinical discussion.

"This is what *happened*" changed to "this is what is *happening*," and therefore, "what are we going to do about it *today*?"

"This guy is in the ER a lot" changed to "Mr. Robinson was in the ER 16 times in the last month and will probably be in another 16 times if we don't do something different."

This reporting increased accountability, as the problems weren't being discussed in hindsight but rather as an active part of the ongoing clinical plan, wherein we were managing current illnesses of the actual *person* in our hospital. This allowed us to address the foundational questions that we in medicine ask ourselves every day and with every patient: "What is the next best step we can take right now to maximize the outcome of this patient?"

It put names and faces to statistics of suffering.

The reporting also put numbers and dollars to problems. It's one thing to be inhumane. We can often deceive ourselves into justifying it, often through blaming patients for their pathologies that we fail to efficiently treat. It's another to be financially wasteful. That's harder to hide from. With the new data, we were able to show the cost of the suffering in our system and the associated recidivism.

The large system-based inefficiencies frustratingly displayed in the 2010 Institute of Medicine report were now filtered down for us, in real time, to the level of the individual patient. The suffering, high cost, and most importantly, opportunity to intervene were all actively in front of us. The pathologies were intense and active. Issues with mental health were highly prevalent, as were the significant social barriers blocking their care. Homelessness was the norm.

I found myself right back in the realm of homeless medicine that I had tried to run from a few years earlier. However, opportunities for improvements were visible everywhere—both at the patient and system levels.

Sometimes, the most innovative thing we can do in medicine is to stop doing the simple things, the fundamentals, so poorly—and finally address the low-hanging fruit efficiently instead of showing off while picking the highest ones.

It turned out that identifying our highest-risk patients though analytics was the easy part of the model. Making the initial connections with these identified patients through proactive outreach, and then subsequently forming trusting clinical relationships, was the real challenge.

The strength of our model was in an initially small group of case managers, and one nurse, who the hospital allowed us to hire. We had a team. The case managers were the leaders and directed patient interactions. That was by design. As the team physician, I followed their lead—not vice versa—as they did the hard work of engaging these patients in the community, on the patients' terms and in their homes, shelters, or streets. They built trust first, and then relationships. They then leveraged these relationships to empower patients to improve their own health.

As part of their plan, the team worked to connect and embed our patients into different community-based organizations and medical clinics to help them achieve long-term success and health.

We definitely found some early low-hanging fruit. In our first year, we identified several uninsured patients with asthma who were intubated in the ICU numerous times in the preceding years, because they couldn't afford the chronic steroid maintenance inhalers needed to control the inflammation in their airways. They were also unable to navigate through the complex application process of the existing free programs within the community. Simply guiding them through this process with close follow-up proved to be successful—and a lot less expensive than repeated patterns of three- to-four day ICU stays.

Preventing exacerbations of diseases is a lot safer, and cheaper, than treating them.

Other opportunities proved to be much harder. We identified numerous patients who were homeless and uninsured in the context of clear disabilities, as defined by Social Security in their *Blue Book*. They were dealing with conditions such as severe cirrhosis, end-stage heart failure, or IQs below 70. (I'm always baffled by how we, as a society, can let the intellectually disabled suffer expensively on the streets and shelters.) Often, it felt like we were arriving too late to effectively divert patients off their trajectories of poor outcomes and mortality. Or, more bothersome, we seemed to be attacking the wrong goals and targets, futilely chasing symptoms while missing the underlying root causes that were hurting and killing our patients.

It still felt like we were often flying blind—which, for me, was disturbingly familiar.

14

BLOODLETTING AND DIRTY HANDS

If we don't understand mechanism in medicine, then we are basically just guessing in our treatments.

Perhaps one of the strangest aspects of the history of American medicine is just how much we've resisted the advancement of knowledge. If you really think about it, before the last 150 years, most of what we did in medicine was truly "quackery." Even at the highest level ... *especially* at the highest level.

On a snowy night in December of 1799, weeks before the turn of the century, George Washington lay ill in his upstairs bedroom at Mount Vernon. He'd spent the past few days outside, working his land in the snow and cold, and had developed a worsening sore throat, fatigue, and eventually breathing issues. As President Washington's symptoms increased, he sent for his long-time friend and personal physician of over 40 years, Dr. James Craik, who subsequently called in two other physicians considered experts at the time. Amidst the faint candlelight, these doctors administered a barrage of different remedies of their time to attempt to stop his clinical deterioration—including enemas, inducing vomiting, creating oral blisters, and the common practice of "bloodletting." In fact, they bled President Washington a total of four times—the last few despite protest from the president's wife, Martha—in hopes they could balance out his fluids and "humors."

While such interventions were considered best practice at the time, they, not surprisingly in hindsight, proved ineffective. President Washington died early on December 14, his body ravaged by what in hindsight was speculated to be bacterial epiglottitis, as well the torture of all the futile medical interventions that were confidently administered to him.[1, 2]

Throughout much of its history, medicine has been practiced in constant violation of our Hippocratic Oath, as the guessing of unknowing and often overly-confident medical providers has proven to be more harmful than simply letting nature and the body, through the filters of billions of years of evolutionary improvements, do their jobs. If an intervention like bloodletting (or hormone replacement with age, or expensive cardiac stents over stable plaques, or back surgeries for pain that will typically resolve by itself) is doing nothing to treat the underlying cause, like infectious epiglottitis, then it has zero benefit and all risk, like bleeding out a patient by removing an estimated 40 percent of their blood volume, as with President Washington.

The science of human biology and pathophysiology that is foundational to medicine is extraordinarily complex. The history of medicine involves recognizing and addressing our ignorance of these complexities as we constantly evolve our field. The reality is that we have often applied more stubborn arrogance than honest intellectual curiosity in this process. Medicine has historically thought highly of itself—so much so that we haven't liked being questioned.

Ignorance mixed with stubborn arrogance is a dangerous combination when trying to better understand that which is complex. It has resulted in greater expense, poorer outcomes, and more than one presidential death.

On July 2, 1881, more than 80 years after President Washington's death, President James Garfield was shot at a train station in Washington, DC. Raised poor and fatherless, Garfield fought political corruption throughout his respected career in Congress before eventually and reluctantly being elected to the highest office in the nation. After just 200 days as president, however, he was the victim of an assassination attempt. He initially survived the two gunshots. One grazed his shoulder. The other was fired point-blank into his back. He was not, however, able to subsequently survive the parade of unwashed hands from the multiple doctors who probed his wounds, one piercing his liver while fumbling around to find the bullet. Even assisted by the new technology of a metal detector developed by Alexander Graham Bell, this team of physicians was never able to dig out the bullet that ultimately proved to be lodged behind his pancreas.

At the time, Luis Pasteur and colleagues in Europe had spent the previous few decades developing the germ theory, arguing that disease was caused by microorganisms that we could not see. Though it was backed by increasingly strong evidence, American medicine at the time resisted this idea, resenting what was perceived as a European theory. This stubborn ignorance resulted in doctor after doctor probing their unwashed hands into President Garfield's wounds—a practice that would definitely be looked down upon in modern medicine. One of the lead physicians, Dr. Bliss, who was an avid opponent of the emerging "European" germ theory at the time, reportedly declared, in opposition to the radical ideas of basic hygiene and handwashing, "the dirtier the better."[3] This claim ultimately proved to be false in the case of President Garfield, who subsequently died, more than two months after he was shot, of intra-abdominal infections resulting from the anti-germ-theory, dirty-hand probing.

In modern medicine, despite all of our amazing advancements and technology, there's evidence that this resistance to change continues. For example, studies have identified what seems to be an extraordinarily long lag time between the discovery of new medical information through research and its actual clinical implementation: 17 years. Seventeen years between when something is discovered and when the average clinician implements it, thereby allowing patients to routinely benefit from the gained knowledge.[4] This statistic supports a high likelihood that a child will never benefit from an advancement in pediatric medicine if it's discovered today.

All of this presents a huge challenge for value-based care, which demands a more rapid pace of change to address the historically costly inefficiencies that are rapidly working to bankrupt our nation. This is especially true as we transform from just treating diseases through medications, tests, and procedures to actually preventing and minimizing poor health outcomes. And, as we pivot our focus to treating root causes of poor chronic health—rather than on just the high-tech and expensive treatment of its symptoms—we will inevitably find ourselves in the communities in which our patients live, with all their social complexities. That is where we will find root causes.

Learning how to address these societal-based root causes can seem overwhelming. We're still very much at the "bloodletting"/"plunging-dirty-hands-into-abdominal-wound" stage when it comes to many aspects of medicine, especially with public health and mental illness. This is definitely the case in homeless medicine, where misunderstood pathologies continue to rage unchecked, hurting and prematurely killing incredible and resilient people.

If it takes 17 years to adapt our preference for oral medications in the treatment of diabetes or accept new concepts such as the germ theory, how long might it take to change the deeply-engrained clinical mis-prioritizations of a multi-trillion-dollar healthcare system that has historically ignored the social determinants driving poor outcomes?

Perhaps if we are deliberate and thoughtful, not as long as we might think.

Knowledge of mechanism is everything, but it doesn't necessarily always have to involve cramming new or complex theories into our already full, routine-focused clinical brains. Sometimes, knowledge is gained by simply opening our eyes to see realities that have always been right in front of us, impacting our daily routines and clinical practices. We just haven't been looking for them.

We've been missing very basic pathologies in medicine, both in our patients and ourselves. If addressed, we can expedite our evolution out of long-standing disparities, inequities, and the expensive, deadly life-expectancy-under-50 mess we find ourselves working through in homeless medicine. This is especially possible if the change is pushed along by rapidly evolving payment models.

For example, in 2016, after numerous meetings and workgroups, our ACO gave up on an effort to expand telemedicine utilization due to lack of provider and payer interest. Between March and June of 2020, telemedicine increased 766 percent nationwide in response to COVID-related lockdowns and social distancing.[5] It helped to maintain patient access and care, and physician payments. This shift took three months, not 17 years.

The business of medicine can evolve quickly when it is incentivized to do so.

PART III
THE TREES

15

KIDS CAMP

Kids Camp was beautiful. Definitely haunted, but beautiful. It was a sharp contrast to the stereotypes I had of New Jersey while growing up in Los Angeles, and served as a testament to its official "Garden State" nickname. Tucked into the base of the mountains in western New Jersey, just miles away from the famous Appalachian Trail, the rolling hills, scattered lakes, and beautiful trees of Kids Camp provided an unexpected contrast to the industrial landscape that shapes most people's views of New Jersey. The camp's 125 acres included a lake, swimming pool, ropes course, farm, and petting zoo. It was the perfect place for kids who lived in the city of Newark's urban landscape to learn about nature while escaping, even for a day, some of the stresses of the city.

On a summer evening in 1999, just a week before I was to start medical school at Georgetown, our camp staff sat under the outside tent where, just hours earlier, hundreds of elementary-school-aged children had eaten lunch. The tent had been effectively transformed from camp lunch-site to party-zone with a few added lights and a keg of beer one of the staff had snuck in. Perhaps feeling nostalgic and reflective, as their time was coming to an end, the college-student staff was tearing up and getting emotional during an impromptu feel-good session that had sprung up around the aforementioned keg. An almost full moon shone brightly on the camp, reflecting off the small lake and providing a beautiful, almost surreal backdrop to the warm, late July evening. The staff recalled their experiences over the summer as it was ending.

The conclusion of the camp felt significant at the time, if not a bit overwhelming. Staff struggled to express their thoughts and put their summer experiences into perspective, yet they didn't necessarily need to, as everybody could relate to one another's stories. A common theme involved being in awe of the children they had worked with over the summer.

It was great to see. I had been nervous about developing a potential guilt complex, as I'd helped to recruit all these students to come to New Jersey. It wasn't an easy summer experience for them.

Eighteen months earlier, I had quit my job with General Electric Medical System in their technical leadership program based in Waukesha, Wisconsin. Not yet confident in my decision to go into medicine after my grandfather's warnings, I'd accepted the job out of college, wanting to experience the business world for a few years before making a definite decision to enter medicine. It was the late 1990s when General Electric, across the multiple sectors of its international conglomerate company, was heavily focused on Six Sigma—a process improvement approach they helped to pioneer that aimed to ensure that 99.99966 percent of manufacturing processes were defect-free. Essentially errorless.

The process fascinated me. The systematic approach of identifying inefficiencies and developing processes to eliminate them was intriguing. While making medical equipment or airplane engines, errors were simply unacceptable, as they could be directly synonymous with death. Even one error in a thousand opportunities would still mean death when building an airplane engine. The process demanded efficiency and accepted nothing less in an effort to minimize cost and optimize outcomes, driven by the necessity of market pressure. I have thought back to this mindset frequently throughout my medical career.

After six months at GE, however, I became more confident

about my desire to attend medical school. Around that time, I received a call from my college friend (and eventual future wife), who was living in Chicago, about an opportunity in New Jersey to work for a nonprofit organization, Kids Corporation, which operated supplemental afterschool and summer education programs for children in Newark.

A few weeks later, we both decided to quit our corporate jobs and move to work at the program's nature camp, located in beautiful Blairstown, New Jersey. Blairstown was famous for two things at the time. First, Blair Academy and their dominant wrestling team that has now won 40 national prep championships, which was awesome. And second, Blairstown was the primary location where the original Friday the 13th horror movie was filmed, which was *not* very awesome—especially with just a few of us living alone in the middle of the woods in the off-season.

We got there in March of 1998 and were thrown immediately into a three-month fire drill, working to recruit the more than 125 students needed to help staff the annual summer programs—which had recently expanded significantly after becoming part of Colin Powell's America's Promise initiative. The organization had been operating its programs for years. Many low-income parents and families depended on the summer sessions Kids Corporation provided, since the programs offered children a safe place to be while continuing their education and "catching up" from the year before. For many parents, this allowed them to work more shifts during the summer.

Kids Camp was developed as a reward for the children attending the main summer programs at the numerous school sites throughout Newark—both public and Catholic. Four days a week, the kids would attend the school programs staffed by the college students staying at Seton Hall University dorms, who assisted the local teachers hired into the program. On a fifth day of the week, the kids would rotate taking the 50-mile bus ride to spend the day at Kids Camp.

The camp had everything necessary to make it an incredible experience for the kids. For many of the children we served, it was the first time they'd really been out in nature—the first time they'd seen a frog, or fished, or taken a nature walk.

We recruited our college staff from both local and national universities. For many of them, it was the first time they had true exposure to the realities of severe poverty and "inner city" issues. However, this was balanced by our college staff who were actually from Newark—many born and raised there. Several of our college staff had actually participated in the summer programs themselves as children.

All our staff, for whatever reason, agreed to come for eight weeks in the summer to earn their $125-per-week AmeriCorps volunteer wage while working with kids who could really benefit from mentorship. Around sixty of these staff members agreed to live at Kids Camp, with its rustic cabins lacking running water and its (relatively clean) outhouses. For most of those college students, this was an opportunity to learn, both from the kids and from each other, and have a lot of fun at night when the kids left for the day. Fun that, as 23-year-old directors, Colleen and I probably contributed way too much to, instead of controlling.

Our staff got real-world exposure outside of their controlled environments of higher institutions of learning, where education was mainly theoretical. Instead of abstract philosophical debates in lecture halls, they received exposure to the real-life manifestations of societal ills, which were playing out amongst the brilliant, smiling, potential-filled kids they worked with. Those realities were often pretty dark and traumatic for the staff to witness (much less for the children to experience).

As the staff taught and grew close to the kids during the summer, they felt at least some comfort in knowing they were doing something to help—no matter how small. But on that night under the tent, the summer—and their time—was coming to an end.

Most were about to return to their secluded institutions of higher learning while the kids would remain behind, continuing their battles of overcoming barriers and hurdles. The staff would no longer be able to help.

This is what they were trying to reconcile on this warm, moonlit summer evening.

One of our staff, Kayla, usually reserved and quiet, started to get emotional about a second-grade girl, Destiny, with whom she had worked through the summer. Kayla spoke of Destiny's brilliance, outgoing personality, and smile—all her positivity that contrasted with the incredible hardships she faced in life.

Destiny's father had been murdered a few years earlier while returning home from work. Her mother suffered from addiction, leading Destiny to live with an overworked aunt who had numerous kids of her own. Kayla was inspired by Destiny's resilience but had serious doubts that she could sustain it over time. It seemed impossible given the constant barrage of hardships that would inevitably keep coming her way. Kayla felt like she was abandoning Destiny.

Cassandra, a staff member who had grown up in the same neighborhood as Destiny and had actually attended the same elementary school, jumped in to try to reassure Kayla. Cassandra was a natural leader and, throughout the summer, had exuded confidence and brilliance that often led to other staff members seeking her advice or input. Going into her junior year at Rutgers in engineering, she seemed mature beyond her years. She pointed out to Kayla that she had made it through circumstances similar to Destiny's.

"I did it. It wasn't easy, but I did it. It's not impossible," Cassandra said in a tone that seemed both reassuring and a bit confrontational.

The normally reserved Kayla shocked everybody when she didn't respond with gratitude for the reassurance that would have kept the feel-good vibes going for the evening. Instead, she replied with a quick and somewhat terse, "Yeah, but you are false advertising."

She didn't mean it as an insult, or as a compliment for that matter; at least I don't think she did. But when she quickly saw people's reactions, she clarified, "You're an exception that makes the impossible seem possible. That's dangerous."

Cassandra quickly replied, "Well, if it was *actually* impossible, how did I *do* it?"—still trying to be reassuring, not antagonistic.

Kayla didn't respond, the conversation ended, and an awkward silence followed.

This unexpected pivot killed the mood of the evening.

It's difficult to see kids suffer. There is universality in the potential and idealism of youth that I think most people can nostalgically look back on and relate to. For most of us, our worldview when we were kids was likely more optimistic and beautiful—often magical—relative to the ones we hold as adults. As kids, most of us, to varying extents, shared an idealism through our dreams, hopes, and imaginations. With age, this often erodes as we witness some of the dark aspects of humanity and their consequences.

But it's important and healthy for kids to share in the idealism of youth. It's tragic when pain, conflict, and stress prevents it or cuts it short. In fact, is there really any greater tragedy than the premature and often violent destruction of the idealism of youth?

The children who were served by the staff in Newark had as much potential and as many dreams as any—dreams and potential that this staff saw daily in the children's smiling, inquisitive faces. That night under the tent, the staff likely, unconsciously or consciously, reflected back on their own childhoods, seeing themselves in this universal potential and eagerness of youth.

We all share a universal desire to develop potential and enjoy life—to experience love, success, and a sense of self-worth. What isn't universal, obviously, is the extent of our opportunities to do so. Nobody ever said life is fair. Everybody must face their own unique challenges and barriers in life. But the number and severity of the constant hardships these kids faced was depressingly eye-opening for our staff. What these kids were being asked to overcome—extreme poverty, loss of parents, drug exposure, violence, trauma—seemed horrifically unfair, because, simply, it *was* horrifically unfair.

Most college staff found this depressing. Kayla, when thinking of Destiny—who defiantly lit up the world around her, despite having to constantly battle through the darkness—was tormented by it.

The energy, determination to help, and love the staff brought daily into the classroom and summer camp was the secret of Kids Corporation's success. It translated into kids who really needed it getting that extra attention, mentorship, and love. The staff created hope. Hope feeds potential. Sometimes brief glimpses of light—and hope to remind you of potential—can be sustaining when you're in the darkness. Potential can be the antidote to darkness, but only if one has a reason to believe in it.

The college staff, while providing this hope—at least to some extent—also came to realize that whatever they provided wasn't nearly enough for many of the kids in their battles. The staff struggled when their time together came to an end.

No matter how determined or energetic the staff was during their short eight-week time at Kids Corporation, most couldn't help but to feel helpless as they realized the extent to which we, as a society, fail to efficiently assist kids in overcoming these barriers. The urgency and efficiency of our efforts couldn't match the severity of harm that was devastating the future potential of these wide-eyed, curious, and energetic children. The children were often being asked to succeed with two hands tied behind their backs, while trying to overcome a non-stop barrage of hurdles being tossed their way as they aged.

For me, during my time at Kids Corporation, the hardest and most disturbing aspect of our job was seeing the realities of these consequences eventually playing out in some of the older kids served by the program. The manifestations of these inequities in childhood opportunities became clear in their divergence of life trajectories. Those "at risk" for bad outcomes were actually starting to manifest those bad outcomes. The damage was already being done, and its impact was accumulating.

A year earlier, Dr. Vincent Felitti and his colleagues released probably the quietest groundbreaking study of all time in a 1998 edition of the *Journal of Preventive Medicine*. In the article, they described the medical and mental health impact of chronic stress on child development. It provided insight into how toxic environments can negatively impact the developing brains and bodies of children

—such as the kids we were working with in Newark. It would describe precisely what we were seeing.

However, it would be years before I, and most others in medicine, paid much attention to it.

Before leaving Kids Camp, through a Robert Wood Johnson Foundation grant, we worked to build and open a medical clinic at the facility to help address the medical conditions we witnessed in the children we served: asthma, poor eyesight (it's tough to learn when you can't see), dental issues, etc. As I started at Georgetown Medical School, I was inspired to address some of the issues I'd seen in Newark. I decided to pursue a career in public health pediatrics.

For the first two years of medical school and the first half of my third-year clinical rotations, I became increasingly confident and excited about my decision to enter pediatrics.

Then I started my inpatient pediatric rotation. One week and three patients later, I changed my mind.

The first patient was a little girl admitted to the hospital due to complications from her progressive and ultimately terminal cancer. She passed away four days later. Watching her suffer, and watching her parents watching her pass away, felt unbearable.

Then there was a burn victim in the ER—an adorable four-year-old boy who had accidentally spilled a boiling pot of water on himself. Seeing him in pain, confused, and scared was agonizing. Upon his admission, I teared up mid-interview with his parents as he cried and moved uncomfortably in his bed.

The straw that broke the camel's back for me was an adorable, chubby two-year-old who came in with a high fever and headache. He needed an immediate lumbar puncture at 2 a.m. to rule out meningitis as a cause for his symptoms. This "don't miss" diagnosis could only be made by assessing spinal fluid to see if it was infected. It took over an hour to successfully complete the procedure that involved placing a needle in his spine to draw out the fluid. For the child, despite all our efforts to console and comfort him as we held him in place for the procedure, it must have felt like torture. As the young resident on the team, I was assigned to give the mom, waiting outside the room and hearing her child's crying, the updates. At first, she was bawling; by the end of the hour, she was screaming. The next day on rounds when we walked into his room, the child immediately hid behind his mother and cowered in fear.

I concluded that it was simply too hard to watch kids suffer. Sick adults at least can understand and comprehend what is going on. Also, a certain amount of age-related health suffering is normal. It's an accepted part of adult medicine, so it's not as traumatizing to see when it occurs. The suffering of a child is just such a stark contradiction to what, ideally, should be the stress-free joy of childhood. It's disturbing.

Really disturbing.

So I ended up, honestly, wimping out and pivoting my career path to internal medicine.

It would be more than 15 years, however, before I realized that ultimately in doing so, I hadn't avoided pediatric suffering and trauma at all. I was just dealing with it in its downstream, messy, and metastatic state.

16

AHA

Dr. Betsey Tilson sat across the table from me in May 2018, at the Panera Bread on the ground floor of WakeMed Hospital.

She was excited, even this early in the morning. A record-setting track star at Dartmouth before attending Johns Hopkins for medical school, her impressive resume contrasted with her genuine humility —all of which circled back to make her a natural leader. A pediatrician, she had dedicated her career to public health.

I'd first met Dr. Tilson soon after I moved to North Carolina, in her role as the local medical director for Medicaid. She later became North Carolina's state medical director, eventually navigating the state through the COVID-19 pandemic and, ultimately, Medicaid expansion. Her enthusiasm around important public health initiatives was always contagious, and her perspectives were always fascinating.

Just months after becoming the state's medical director, she had agreed to meet with me as a favor after I had called her a week earlier flustered and confused.

Early with our hotspotter model, we noticed, and proved, that our hospital was full of patients truly there due to unmet social needs, having nowhere else to go and no social support system to help when they felt sick or unsafe. This was especially true for our most vulnerable patients—both from a medical and mental health perspective.

Our ER beds were often their last option. Out of necessity, our clinical approach with these patients increasingly focused on addressing the gaps in these social safety nets by getting into the community with them. There, we could help these patients navigate the chaos they were battling.

As we did so, however, we noticed something fascinating: It was a two-way street. In the community, we discovered our local social services were filled with clients who were there mainly for unmet medical and behavioral health needs. Our homeless shelters were full of disabled residents who couldn't work due to medical conditions. Our jails and prisons were our community's largest mental health facilities. Our ambulances were heavily utilized by residents with no other options or access to care. We saw clearly the vast, dangerous, and expensive disconnect between our local social services and health systems—with patients/residents suffering as they volleyed between them.

Social services and community-based organizations routinely failed to impact their most challenging clients needing help. The complexities of the requirements, follow-ups, and applications required to engage their services could easily overwhelm clients who were just trying to survive on a day-to-day basis, burdened by their medical and mental health issues. Clients with severe and persistent mental health issues were routinely being blocked, barred, or trespassed away from services. They often had no choice but to seek the help, safety, or shelter they knew they could find in our healthcare safety nets, if even for a brief period. Once in our safety net, we failed to effectively manage the pathologies that landed them there in the first place.

We knew this pattern of mutual failures was expensive. We were inefficiently hemorrhaging taxpayer money. But to date, our hotspotter model had only captured the health cost side of the equation. If we were to truly appreciate the potential benefits of more efficient interventions, we needed to calculate the social cost as well.

To successfully advocate for sustainable changes aimed at closing this expensive gap between medicine and social services, we needed our political and healthcare leaders to understand the financial implications of our shortcomings. We had to shift the discourse away from simply idealistic, feel-good arguments. To secure support for the broader legislative reforms needed to make taxpayer-funded community health initiatives more efficient, we had to develop a business case. This would require buy-in from across the community.

Fortunately, as we were learning and gaining experience in our medical hotspotter model, our local Wake County's Board of Commissioners were simultaneously building "health in all policies" strategies that aligned with our population health efforts in medicine. Both sides of the gap were already paying attention to each other. Throw in the local IT infrastructure found in the Research Triangle, and then add the buy-in of our other two local health systems, Duke and UNC, who were forging through their own early population efforts in a state without Medicaid expansion, and we were positioned—as well as any community in the country—to address this historic gap between medicine and social services.

In 2017, Wake County developed the Population Health Task Force to do just that.

The large group of leaders from all sectors of Wake County—healthcare, judicial, government, education, faith, and community-based organizations—would fill the Wake County Commissioners' boardroom. Discussions revolved around improving community coordination and ensuring that all residents could achieve health.

Specifically, this task force discussed and came to better understand the complex interactions between social needs and health, and the resulting impact on societal costs. We learned from the best practices of other communities working on similar efforts. We heavily focused on one model from Silicon Valley that utilized shared databases to calculate the predicted costs of their "familiar faces" in an effort to prioritize the limited availability of housing. Often, the annual costs of these individuals would routinely be $200,000 to $300,000.[1] The models looked at the potential cost reductions associated with prioritizing these individuals into housing.

Around the large oak boardroom table, our community discussed how to effectively bridge the historical gap between medicine and social services—a chasm where preventable and expensive human suffering resided. What sort of legislation, policies, and strategies were needed? How could we use data to prioritize efforts and then track outcomes in a way that could adapt and evolve models efficiently? In order to truly capture the complete return on investment of these interventions, such models would require "whole person analytics" to capture not only hospital utilization, but also jail days, homeless shelter stays, EMS visits, etc.

Our efforts with the county's task force were divided into three focus areas, depicted as a pyramid.

The bottom tier represented "healthy communities"—how to support the overall well-being of all county residents. This would involve such infrastructure as park systems, trails, and public health policies. The middle tier was "at-risk vulnerable populations"— groups at risk for poor outcomes, and potentially for becoming our "future familiar faces." The committee eventually selected vulnerable children with trauma to be the focus area of this group. And the top tier was the "familiar faces"—our most vulnerable, sickest, and most expensive residents. These were individuals with frequent interactions with our healthcare systems, social service programs, and law enforcement—who were suffering tremendously and at a high cost.[2] As these were the individuals typically being engaged by our hospital's hotspotter model, I was asked to co-chair the Familiar Face committee.

As we discussed priorities, a consensus grew to focus many of our efforts "upstream," accompanied by constant conversation around what quickly had become a popular buzzword: adverse childhood events, or ACEs. As defined by the CDC, ACEs are "... potentially traumatic events that occur in childhood (0–17 years). Examples include experiencing violence, abuse or neglect; witnessing violence in the home or community; or having a family member attempt or die by suicide. Also included are aspects of the child's environment that can undermine their sense of safety, stability or bonding. Examples can include growing up in a household with substance abuse problems, mental health problems, instability due to parental separation or household members being in jail or prison."[3] (See Appendix for ACE Screening Tool.)

The interest locally at the time was largely due to an incredible 2016 documentary, *Resilience*, directed by James Redford, based on that 1998 study by Dr. Felitte and the work that Dr. Nadine Burkett in California was doing to clinically address ACEs in vulnerable pediatric populations. The documentary was shown a few times locally for the public. People were excited. Conversations around ACEs not only drove discussion around our "middle tier of the pyramid" strategies, but they had started to dominate "entire pyramid" conversations.

My initial reaction of intellectual curiosity quickly turned to frustration.

I had spent my career "downstream," working with a population often forgotten or overlooked. A lot of incredible charities and efforts focused on helping children, but there weren't as many interested in adults suffering from severe, persistent, and chronic homelessness. Societal sympathy for kids suffering from trauma inevitably turns to judgment and blame as they age into no-longer-adorable adults, demonstrating trauma's often messy and scary manifestations. And here was the task force talking about "moving upstream" —focusing on preventing damage instead of dealing with the expensive chaos that already existed.

In theory, prevention was super. I was all for it. But there should always be a sense of urgency to control the pain and poor outcomes immediately in front of us. Failing to do so is expensive and often results in the human suffering and death that I was tired of seeing daily.

Frustrated, I reached out to Dr. Tilson to gain more context. Fortunately, she was more than willing to help. She clearly saw the link between chronic pediatric stress and the long-term outcomes mentioned in the original ACE study. As a self-proclaimed "geek," she had already dived in and studied ACEs and the impact of trauma—not only at the neuroanatomic level but down to the DNA and molecular level. As North Carolina's medical director, she had started to advocate for the long-term health benefits of better recognizing and addressing ACEs. She agreed to meet me for breakfast at the hospital's Panera Bread early that May morning to discuss this further.

And she brought PowerPoint slides. She only had three.

The first—titled "How Early Experiences Alter Gene Expression and Shape Development"—was a slide she'd adapted from the Harvard Center on the Developing Child. It demonstrated how external experiences such as stress, nutrition, and environmental toxins trigger signals between our brain's neurons that launch the production of proteins. These proteins—designed to regulate the actual expression of our genes—either attract or repel enzymes that will then either add or remove markers controlling how much a certain gene is expressed. Essentially, this entire process will either turn on or off a gene, "thereby shaping how brains and bodies develop." The stress hormones turn *on* genes in the parts of the brain that control emotion or "reaction." However, in the parts of the brain that involve contemplation or reflection, it does the exact opposite—closing down DNA expression.[4]

This made sense. When the body is forced into survival mode in response to significant stress, it will prioritize developing the brain regions designed to help it do so—not those focused on the luxury of higher learning or cognition. A brain under constant stress prioritizes basic survival while sacrificing cognitive and social development. The slide showed the mechanisms behind this, down to the basics of genetic expression. Stress can't actually change a person's genes. It can, however, affect how genes are expressed and controlled.

She moved on to her next slide, illustrating the typical clinical symptoms of these stress-induced neuroanatomic changes. The prefrontal cortex is one of the deprioritized, reflective parts of the brain where stress leads to neuronal loss; it's involved with thought, memory, and risk processing. The impact of stress on this part of the brain can help explain the findings of studies that show trauma in childhood results in more academic struggles and less achievement in school.[5] The prefrontal cortex is also responsible for "cognitive flexibility"—safely and appropriately adapting behavior based on one's changing environment. Poor prefrontal cortex development can also result in difficulty with change, problem-solving, multitasking, and flexibility or ability to respond to feedback. Finally, impaired prefrontal cortex function can result in poor impulse control and struggles with prospective memory. This includes remembering to do a planned action in the future, something we use constantly to help us stay organized and functional: taking medications, showing up on time for an appointment, or efficiently managing daily tasks.

Constant stress, and its associated impact on genetic expression, results in the underdevelopment of another part of the brain, the hippocampus, which helps to support memory and learning—demonstrating another link between childhood stress and academic struggles. Development of higher and theoretical learning may not be a luxury one is afforded if they are constantly "running from the bear." The hippocampus also helps a person interpret threats and put them into appropriate context.

The slide also illustrated the reactive parts of the brain that are "turned on" by stress. These regions are responsible for processing emotions, instincts, and survival. It focused on the amygdala, the part of the brain responsible for "immediate emotional processing." When this gets hypertrophied, or over-developed, it results in over-reactivity, fear, and anxiety. Essentially, the brain becomes easily triggered—always ready to react, to survive.

Her third and final slide showed MRI images of children who

suffered from neglect and chronic toxic stress compared to ones who did not. The brains of children who suffered from severe trauma were smaller and underdeveloped compared to those without trauma. The difference was stark. This slide was the most disturbing, pulling back from the molecular and genetic levels to clearly demonstrate the physical and neuroanatomic consequences of ACEs. It provided a bird's-eye view of the damage from the storms.

The impact of stress on the developing brain occurs early—really early—highlighting the importance of employing strategies not only at the pediatric level, but even in the prenatal period when the brain is rapidly growing.

(Years later, in 2022, I would give a grand rounds presentation for the University of Texas Pediatrics Department on this topic—specifically on trauma-informed interventions in unhoused pregnant women. We discussed how there's perhaps no greater public health intervention than optimizing the physical and mental health in women experiencing high-risk pregnancies in the context of addiction, mental illness, trauma, and/or homelessness.)

As I sat that morning in the hospital restaurant listening to Dr. Tilson explain all of this, my head spun. She was describing so much of what had been blurred or mysterious to me over the years. It was truly a *Sixth Sense* moment, putting into context so much of what I'd failed to recognize in my patients over the years.

As she finished, she emphasized: "It is *all* trauma. We *have* to do better."

One one hand, this improved understanding brought relief. On the other, a sense of hopelessness settled in as I realized just how engrained, anatomical, and biological the barriers to health had been for the patients I had cared for over the years. I thought back to not only the kids we served in Newark, but also so many of the patients I'd worked with over the years. I guessed that our patients who suffered from homelessness would have a higher prevalence of historic ACEs than the general population.

It wasn't hard to quickly confirm my supposition.

I found that in the general population, 3 to 5 percent of people suffered from four or more adverse childhood events.

In those who suffered from homelessness, that rate was 54 percent.[6] (In a study our team would later perform at a local Raleigh substance abuse treatment program with a group of 144 men and women experiencing homelessness, that number would be 74 percent.)

This disparity clarified the vague references we (or at least I) had made about "rough childhoods"—without really appreciating the impact of those childhoods nor the mechanisms of their damage.

I tried to imagine the incomprehensible nightmares of youth that most patients who suffered from chronic homelessness had lived through. Each tragedy progressively darkening their world, and as more of life's roads became blocked, their optimism and associated joy of youth prematurely vanishing. There is a violent dehumanization inherent in many of the ACEs—a complete disregard for the child.

How tragic and confusing must it be to try to process being a victim of this as a child? How must it feel to suffer in a world that can't see or help what's happening to them? How deflating and painful must it be when any inconsistent sympathy and support they may have received in youth inevitably turns into consistent judgment and blame as they age?

Society's inherent sympathy for the suffering child quickly and predictably dissolves as that child's suffering evolves into the messy and often ugly downstream manifestations of trauma. Stereotypes take over. Societal sympathy has a small and definite window that will quickly flip to blame as victims of ACEs grow older. The inherent, God-given beauty and potential that radiates from kids dims from view with age, even though it's still there underneath the scars of time, trauma, and chaos.

It's the same child, individual, soul, and human deep inside, battling through the suffering. We just become blind to their humanity—literally, as I would learn later. We become too superficially focused on the scars.

The violent acts of dehumanization inherent in ACEs plant the seeds for the brutal dehumanization of blame and bias against its victims, which metastasize through adulthood and even across generations. Trauma begets more trauma; it's a deadly positive feedback cycle.

For years, I'd been disturbed by the mortality data in homeless populations. That data around the prevalence of childhood trauma in adults experiencing homelessness was just as haunting as the mortality data on the other end.

It turns out the two are intrinsically linked.

Homeless adults die, on average, decades before the general population. A study in 2013 led by one of my former colleagues at BHCHP, Dr. Travis Baggett, demonstrated the causes driving this early mortality. It isn't just related to overdoses or addiction. They have a higher prevalence of heart disease. Of cancer. Of deadly infections.[7]

I'd always just kind of chalked this up to some nebulous, destiny-of-doom, horrible-luck version of Murphy's Law that sadly impacted our patients—a view that I think is common and results in a lot of shoulder shrugging and defeatism. *What are we going to do? The cards are just hopelessly stacked against them.* Obviously, this is not too scientific and in direct contrast to the Occam's Razor theory in medicine: One simple cause, a unifying diagnosis, can often explain multiple symptoms. We often get so distracted managing the complexities of the manifestations of disease that we forget to identify and address the disease itself. Instead of bad luck here, bad luck there—an early heart attack here and a random cancer there—what is the root cause? Coincidence stops being coincidence when it keeps happening. "Bad luck" is not an acceptable medical explanation.

It turns out that the pathologic consequences of trauma don't remain confined in childhood. They set the foundation for poor health outcomes for the future. The four or more ACES that the majority of the homeless population has suffered increase the risk of 7 out of 10 leading causes of death in America. People who experienced four or more ACES as children also experience a four- to six-fold increase in the prevalence of diabetes, cancer, heart disease, asthma, and COPD as adults. They have a 15-times higher rate of suicide and 12-times higher rate of behavioral health challenges.[8,9]

Chronic stress is pathologic for the entire body, not just for the brain. This makes sense given its physiologic mechanism: Stress is nonspecific, with a hormonal cascade that's designed to quickly blast and activate the entire body. It's intuitive that its chronic, toxic form would be nonspecific in its physiologic damage.

The reasons behind the early mortality we were seeing in our populations seemed to directly point back to those early childhood traumas. The suffering, and its associated stress and negative impact on the body, were often constant throughout their lives—from start to finish. The physiologic trajectories our patients were placed on as children were often stubbornly pointed toward where they ended up. Their suffering was almost inevitable—physiologically and neuroanatomically hardwired.

Prevention is always the best medicine. If an ounce of prevention is worth a pound of cure, a pound of prevention is worth a ton of cure—especially when the disease is as dangerous and confusing as the physiologic damage of severe trauma.

The damage seemed to be almost metastatic and "end-stage" for so many of my patients by the time I was caring for them. So focusing our efforts on preventing or minimizing its harm in the first place made sense. I understood that push to move upstream. I jumped on board.

The first thing I did after the meeting with Dr. Tilson was call Dr. Rasheeda Monroe, the medical director for WakeMed pediatrics at the time.

"Have you ever heard of ACEs?!" I excitedly asked her.

I'm pretty sure she sighed. … I'm almost positive I heard a sigh—a well-disguised sigh, but still a sigh.

"Yes," she said.

17

THE CURMUDGEON

In medicine, we often do not communicate efficiently between our large, typically siloed departments.

I spent the next few weeks learning about the work that Dr. Monroe, her colleague Dr. Carrie Dow-Smith, and their pediatric department had been doing to address adverse childhood events ... in their medical silo ... just next to mine ... in the same system ... for years. Not only had she heard of ACEs, but they had been innovating and researching family-based interventions in their clinic through grant funding. Their work focused on supporting the caregivers of the children who were suffering from trauma to help alleviate these children's overall stress levels. Their program was serving hundreds of families annually. She and Dr. Dow Smith had also been advocating for years to develop trauma-informed education for hospital medical provider, so more could benefit from the aha moment I'd had in the hospital cafeteria that morning with Dr. Tilson.

Over the next few months, I quickly became convinced of the following: In true population health models, there's *nothing* more important than a focus on pediatric mental health—and therefore pediatric trauma, if we are to efficiently address root causes. From a cross-generational perspective, there is no greater potential return on investment than in doing so, both financially and in reducing human suffering. But these results come over the *long term*, which is exactly why the opportunity was largely being ignored.

The payment models of accountable care organizations, and value-based care in general, are determined by year-to-year numbers, paralleling the focus of insurance companies and hospital partners. We must hit annual metrics around cost and quality, so we focus on those numbers with the highest potential for immediate impact. Annual cost-savings calculations are based on our performance compared to the prior years. The design and its associated metrics and incentives focus on immediate results—not necessarily on long-term health or preventive measures, where any resulting cost savings wouldn't be realized for years, perhaps generations.

Better addressing pediatric trauma, improving nutrition at school, supporting systems for children with incarcerated parents—there's a huge potential financial impact of such programs that could improve a child's long-term health trajectories. Yet these are more theoretical and future-based, and therefore easy to ignore as we obsess with the more immediate cost of the patients we're being held accountable for *this year*. So instead we focus on blood sugar control, vaccination rates, reducing ER visits, and our $100,000-plus-annual-cost patients—the "top 1 percent." These factors are more tangible, as they're immediate. More doable, and ultimately, while important, probably less impactful and meaningful.

Once again, even early on in the new value-based care models, we had become comfortable in the downstream; we had relatively little understanding about the upstream. We were too distracted to listen to those who had forged their way up there tell us about what they discovered.

But even through this haze of misdirected priorities, the potential was intuitive enough that it was impossible to ignore—especially with a better grasp of the science behind it. If we worked strategically, scientifically, and innovatively to do our best to assist a child who suffered from ACEs—redirecting these trajectories away from their downstream manifestations—the resulting impact, both in terms of human suffering and societal cost, could be enormous, even if it was hard to appreciate with our year-to-year mindset.

From an ACO perspective, we decided if there was any group that could work to address ACEs, it would be our ACO, as one-third of our 400-plus primary care physicians were pediatricians. Our pediatric providers at the time were already attesting to their increased struggles in dealing with pediatric mental health in the context of social media and other societal factors.

I asked Dr. Tilson to lead a dinner lecture with our providers.

More than 100 local pediatricians attended a meeting in one of our hospital's large conference rooms. Dr. Tilson presented the same slides she had shown me. We also showed the *Resilience* documentary, with discussions led by Dr. Tilson, Dr. Monroe, Dr. Dow-Smith, and others.

Many attendees had already heard of ACEs; some had not. Several had aha and *Sixth Sense* moments. Pediatricians discussed with excitement how this could impact their practices and their patients.

But there is always that one curmudgeon in the house. The contrarian. That night, it was a family physician who had been serving the community for years. After the meeting was finished, he made his way through the other providers who were staying to ask questions of the speakers.

As he strolled up to me, he looked neither inspired nor aha'ed.

"Well, that was complete bullshit. What the hell are we supposed to do about any of this?" he blurted out.

By this time, I'd found it a certainty that no matter how well a presentation went or how intuitive the topic was, there would always be interactions like this. They were inevitable—including on this night. With more than 400 primary providers in our ACO, even if the dissenters were a small minority, they would still exist. However, this one surprised me, as this provider was involved with our ACO committees and clinical workgroups. He was engaged. He definitely wasn't a cheerleader, but he wasn't a narcissist contrarian either.

Even more surprising about his comment was that at the end of the documentary, it described outcomes of successful, community-based interventions—ones the speaker's panel had also discussed after the film. Had he not seen and heard what I'd just witnessed?

"Didn't you see the end of the movie?" I asked, somewhat frustrated. "Didn't you hear the discussions afterward?"

He shot back, "There will always be ACEs in the community. It's beyond our control. We can't be distracted into thinking we can do anything about them. We are too damn busy." He then turned and walked away, but not before muttering one last time "Complete waste of an evening."

A few weeks later, I was discussing potential grant opportunities with Dr. Monroe and Dr. Dow-Smith. The basic idea was this: Our hotspotter model worked "downstream" in the chaos, often addressing the suffering and expensive consequences of historical ACEs. As we continued to work at better managing and addressing the chaos, we would build analytics to help capture and quantify the associated cost avoidance. We could then quantify these savings and reinvest a portion upstream, toward prevention, through potential grant matches. This cross-generational design could make everything more cohesive for us, and for our potential funders.

Better manage the chaotic downstream manifestations of trauma while working to prevent them upstream. That's *exactly* what medicine should work to do. Improve our stage-four breast cancer treatments while simultaneously improving our mammogram techniques and rates to optimize prevention. Develop innovative end-stage heart failure interventions while working to identify and treat early risk factors. More ounces of prevention to better avoid the painful, expensive, and often unsuccessful pounds of cure. So why not apply this principle to the issue of ACEs and their later consequences?

Better treat symptoms while we work to prevent root causes.

I explained to Dr. Monroe and Dr. Dow-Smith that, for me and our "downstream" team, we'd gain motivation by knowing that the calculated cost savings of our success could help fund preventive efforts designed to help divert kids from the paths of the dark realities we worked in on a daily basis. Once on those paths, it seemed almost impossible to get anyone off. The trajectories we were trying to redirect were too stubborn.

"From a neuroanatomy perspective, the damage is done. In many of our patients, we're stuck trying to deal with the broken that can't be fixed," I lamented.

They both looked at me, confused, similar to how I must have looked at the post-awesome-talk curmudgeon. I knew right away I'd likely said something stupid; I just, for the life of me, had no idea what.

"Yes it can. That is the whole point," Dr. Dow-Smith replied.

The neuroanatomic damage could be addressed—just not through our modern-day bloodletting.

18

NEUROPLASTICITY

Mary sat across from me in my downtown Raleigh clinic. Her face was embarrassed as she struggled to find her words. She came by herself, not wanting family or friends to assist her.

She teared up as she continued to struggle. She became frustrated when I tried to jump in and "help" by trying to guess the words she couldn't get out. She was a lawyer—a good one—and had built her career around her skills of articulation. She'd been blindsided a few weeks earlier by a stroke despite having no real risk factors.

Mary was sitting on the couch reading with her husband when it happened—initially painless and subtle. She noticed she couldn't communicate with her husband, as the words she wanted to say were out of reach. "A complete nightmare—I felt trapped," she would later describe. Terrified, she tried to get up to call 911; that's when she noticed her right-sided weakness. An MRI would later demonstrate that a random clot had closed the superior branch of her middle cerebral artery despite all her other blood vessels being found entirely disease-free.

In my clinic that day, Mary struggled with her new expressive aphasia. She knew what she wanted to say to the world; she just couldn't actually say it, which had always been her specialty. She was much more focused on this aphasia than on her right arm and leg weakness. Mary looked paralyzed and trapped. This was a horrible contrast to the annual physicals I'd usually see her for, wherein we'd celebrate her good health and lifestyle habits and talk about how she could continue maximizing them moving forward.

As we reviewed her care plan that day, I encouraged her to go "all-in" with the speech and physical therapy—and to continue struggling through these conversations. Getting pissed off was her brain working to adapt and heal.

"Fight … like … hell!" she stammered with significant effort and tears in her eyes just before leaving that day.

Almost three months later, she returned to my clinic. When I noticed she was on my schedule, I was nervous to see her progress. I walked in; she was sitting in her chair in formal work attire. She stood up, walked over, stuck out her right hand, and with a firm handshake and a huge smile, effortlessly and without a stutter said, "Can we make it quick? I have to be back at work in 30 minutes for a lunch meeting."

Neuroplasticity is awesome. Reason number 2,327,657 why our human bodies are incredible beyond our current comprehension.

Neuroplasticity is the concept that our nervous system can continuously change in response to the environment. Nerves can shrink and die or expand and increase connections. In cases like Mary's (especially in the first three months after a stroke), or in a child who has suffered abuse, or in the 50-year-old patient chronically living on the streets and still battling the trauma of their childhood, the final answer is never: "The damage is done." Our brains are constantly changing, growing, and adjusting to the world around them. There's always potential in our neuroanatomy.

This is what both Dr. Curmudgeon and I forgot, or chose not to focus on, in our reflexive pessimism. The brain has the ability to heal itself and adapt to its environments and injuries. As providers, our job is to facilitate the healing processes for our patients to the "best of our abilities"—or, at the very least, to "do no harm."

Yet despite this being a foundational principle of the Hippocratic Oath, it seems like we violate it on a daily basis, both on an individual and a population-based level, in our interactions with patients who have mental illness and histories of trauma.

In order to better treat our patients' medical issues, we need to address the behavioral health pathologies that exacerbate them. To do this, we have to become much better at addressing underlying historical trauma. Perhaps this is the formula that can reverse engineer better treatments for the downstream complications killing our patients.

However, healthcare providers, above everything else, are human. The personal interaction between a provider and patient is at the foundation of medicine. Pathologies can be two-sided, occurring on both sides of this interaction. In medicine, we often see the splinter in the eye of our patient while hypocritically missing the beam in our own.

PART IV
THE FOREST

19
REFLEXIVE DEHUMANIZATION

Alcohol can sometimes be a truth serum.
A few years ago, my wife, Colleen, threw out the one oversized suit I had worn since medical school that she mistakenly thought made me look like MC Hammer, parachute pants and all. I still loved it. She did not. So, it got tossed. I then bet her I could find another suit under $100 on Amazon, and it would look amazing.

I won that bet (at least according to me). It's still the only suit I own. I typically wear it about once a year, as we do not attend (and/or get invited to?) many fancy events.

This was one of those nights when I excitedly got to strut it out.

We were at a fundraising gala in a large ballroom. As it was getting later in the evening, and with music starting as people headed toward the dance floor, the initial, more formal conversations were increasingly evolving toward much louder, more uninhibited conversations—about $100 Amazon suits, but about many other things as well.

In relaxed social situations, especially if drinks are involved, people will often let their guard down and reveal true beliefs. In a world of cautious smiling/nodding aimed at conforming to the norms of an increasingly politically correct world, this can result in more honest conversations—good and bad.

The danger of an overly politically correct world is that it's often superficial. Real personal actions are driven by actual, inherently held beliefs, not by obligatory acknowledgments made to avoid anticipated scorn or judgment. An overreliance on political correctness can disguise these inherent beliefs and their associated actions and behaviors. It can also stifle dialogue, providing a cover to inaction and a widening gap between our societal words and actions.

As part of a burnout-prevention strategy, I try to avoid bringing my work home with me. I won't discuss it much at home with family or socially with friends. People who know me, however, are generally aware that I work in "homeless medicine" and are supportive, albeit sometimes confused. The most common reaction is typically something along the lines of "thank God somebody is doing it" and associated expressions of gratitude. All of which is awesome and usually very genuine.

However, you get a couple of drinks in people, and that's when the real questions and conversations will often start.

At the event, toward the end of the night, I met the father of one of my son's soccer teammates. We were both trying to avoid being pulled onto the dance floor by our wives, who eventually just gave up and started dancing by themselves. He was a nice guy who I had never really spoken to previously, although our wives were friends. He worked locally in Raleigh and was active in his church.

Our conversation revolved around his work for a while. It then evolved into his frustration around some changes made in his son's youth soccer league, which resulted in what he believed was unfair team placement for his child on a lower team—or something like that. He was pretty revved up about it before he pivoted to other topics, going to the familiar "what do you do for work?" question.

He was interested and very engaged as I told him. He referenced some of the work done by his church with homeless outreach, which he'd been part of. After a few minutes, he started to tell me about a man near his work who had been panhandling on the same street corner for almost a year—always in the same clothes and always at the same location.

"He always holds one of two different cardboard signs that he alternates between," he described. "And he typically talks to himself loudly, which makes him seem a bit intimidating."

With some frustration, and genuine honesty, he described his struggles with feeling compassion for this individual, and for other individuals experiencing homelessness who he had encountered near his work. He wanted to and felt like he should—he *knew* that he should—but he just couldn't. This made him feel like a hypocrite when he was at church or teaching his kids. Frustrated, he summed it up: "My big issue is this, and I don't mean to sound like a jerk, but it's just how I feel: God helps those who help themselves. Perhaps if they spent less time in self-pity and complaining and just got a job, they wouldn't be homeless. They have the time."

By that point in the evening, he'd likely drunk a bit too much to appreciate the irony of complaining about the complaining by those suffering from homelessness after he'd just complained about the grave, youth-soccer-related injustices he and his family had to endure. These seemed likely much less burdensome, relatively speaking, than homelessness.

However, what he said was very familiar.

Throughout the years, I've known good people who admit to the same difficulty in feeling empathy for people experiencing homelessness. This is especially true in areas where homelessness has been skyrocketing, such as my home state of California. The more people see it, especially the more it impacts their lives in potentially negative ways, the less sympathy they feel. Like this very authentically nice, church-going, family-orientated man, people seem to be genuinely bothered by their inability to feel empathy, as it runs contrary to their self-perception of being, hopefully, kind and caring people.

They're perplexed by this gap between what they know they should feel and what they actually *do* feel. They know they should be feeling something they are not—and are unsure why this is the case.

Coming out of my medical training, I now realize I had shared the same perceptions and stereotypes around homelessness. In fact, they were the main barrier to me initially considering a position with BHCHP. I wanted to work with and treat patients who "wanted to help themselves." The idea underlying this, which I realized later in hindsight, was that I viewed homelessness as self-inflicted.

The fact that all of this runs contrary to the core principles of humanitarianism—which for most of us helps guide our personal values—doesn't sit well with us. This is especially the case with those who consider themselves to be religious.

The call to love and not judge others is almost universal among world religions. Compassion is one of the most used words in the *Quran*. Loving, while expecting nothing in return, is a central theme of Hinduism. One of the core commandments of Judaism is: **"Love your neighbor as yourself"** (Leviticus 19:18). None of these teachings are qualified with an out-clause of "… but only when it's easy." It would make our lives much easier if they were, but they aren't. In fact, most religious teachings emphasize the need to love, *especially* when it is hard. All seem to warn us of a human tendency to judge others and implore us not to act on it. Jesus's warning in the Bible is perhaps one of the most direct: "Judge not and you shall not be judged" (Luke 6:37).

When we meet somebody, we have no idea about their history. About their upbringing. About how their environment interacted with them, and they with their environment, and how it all affected and influenced them. Luckily, we don't need to figure all of that out. Our job is, in theory, much easier we just have to reflexively love.

So why is this so hard to actually do?

The work of Dr. Lasana Harris and his colleagues might provide the answer.

―――

Before going overseas to teach and research at University College London, Dr. Harris was a social neuroscience professor and researcher at Duke University. The field of social cognition is fascinating. In recent years it has evolved from the historically social, observation-driven field of psychology to a more advanced understanding through imaging of the brain to study how it functions. Through an improved knowledge of neuroanatomy, the field seeks to improve our knowledge of exactly how our brain works to direct human behaviors. While many in the field are working to learn how to manipulate and addict the human mind through social media, short videos, and clickbait, Dr. Harris has dedicated his career to studying how we can use this information to improve our humanity—and avoid the violent and dangerous traps that we've consistently fallen into throughout history in our human interactions.

In many ways, medicine is still in the "Dr. Craik, bloodletting stage" in our understanding of how the human brain works. Pioneers like Dr. Harris are working hard to pull us out of our ignorance. His research attempts to understand the neuroanatomic pathways underlying human interactions and relationships. He has a special interest in when these "go wrong"—specifically understanding how advanced societies tolerate the suffering of, or even human atrocities against, certain populations. How can human brains tolerate and accept unimaginable evils such as genocide and persecution of fellow humans, often with such blatant hypocrisy?

For example, a small, red-tile-roofed church was built directly over the male dungeons in Ghana's Cape Coast Castle, a major center for the transatlantic slave trade. In the 18th century, parishioners could look down during their religious services to witness the unimaginable suffering, pain, and death of the slave captives held in the well-documented, harsh conditions of overcrowding and poor sanitation. They could observe the courtyard where these slaves were forced through the Door of No Return—the final exit point for millions of enslaved Africans before boarding the ships that would take them to the Americas. Most never returned to their homeland.[1]

On Sunday mornings in the late 1930s and early 1940s, the majority of residents in Nazi Germany woke up and went to church. This included 40 million Protestants and 20 million

Catholics[2] walking past Jewish neighbors and the daily demonstrations of the Holocaust playing out in front of them.

How could such societies tolerate and accept such dehumanization, persecution, and death of genocide? The same question could be asked of the Hutu ethnic majority during the Rwanda genocide against the Tutsi.

How could slave traders and owners reconcile their Christianity with their acts of daily violence against, and disregard for, humanity?

On the world's battlefields throughout history, how have people pulled the trigger, or dropped the bombs, knowing their actions would result in life-changing trauma for sons, daughters, mothers, fathers, siblings, and spouses of the strangers they targeted—with unimaginable loss, grief, and trauma creating new ACEs?

In 2011, Dr. Harris coauthored a study with Princeton researcher, Dr. Susan Fiske, that was designed to understand the science of dehumanization. This particular study focused specifically on homelessness. As they explained in the introduction to their study, "People talk to their computers and their cars, imputing intent and other mental states, but they avoid eye contact with the homeless panhandler in the subway, shutting out his mind and hence his humanity." They sought to better understand how, and therefore why, this occurs.

In their study published in the *Journal of Psychology*, they placed Princeton undergraduate students in a functional MRI machine that assessed brain activity through changes in blood flow. They briefly flashed pictures of people representative of different groups of society—a "female college student and male American firefighter … a businesswoman and rich man … an elderly man and disabled woman … and a female homeless person and male drug addict." What they found: The area of the brain involved with social interactions and humanization, the medial prefrontal cortex, lit up when visualizing every picture *besides* those of the "addict" and "homeless person."[3] Instead, the area of the brain involved with disgust, the anterior insula, lit up with activity.

The study fascinated me—and offered the greatest aha moment in my medical journey of working with homeless populations.

On a larger scale, it provided understanding for questions around tolerance and even support for human atrocities that Dr. Harris and Dr. Fiske were seeking. As Dr. Harris explained: "When we encounter a person, we usually infer something about their minds. Sometimes, we fail to do this, opening up the possibility that we do not perceive the person as fully human."[4] Hitler calling Jews "vermin" or "rats," or Rwanda's propaganda depicting the Tutsi as "cockroaches," facilitated the dehumanization necessary for their populations to tolerate the horrors of genocide.

For me personally, the study helped to explain the foundations of society's frequent indifference toward the suffering of those experiencing homelessness. It provided the neurobiological explanation for dehumanization, from the soccer dad's inability to feel empathy for the man at the street corner to our collective and apparently reflexive societal response to homelessness. It was the source of the pain that Peter articulated so well, years before he gave me the "I Love Boston" teddy bear key chain, about what he found to be the most painful aspect of being homeless: "Nobody treats you like a normal person. Some will treat you with pity, most with disdain, but nobody treats you like a normal person." And it was reflected in Joanne's quote at the grade school lecture: "The hardest part was not feeling hungry or cold, or not knowing where I would sleep, but rather feeling invisible to others. Sometimes people would not even look at me, even if I was hurt ... as if I wasn't even human."

As my very first Hostage US client told me, "There is no greater pain than that of being treated as less than human." This is a message I have heard multiple times from patients I have served over the years.

Our reflexive social reaction to people experiencing homelessness typically isn't sympathy or concern, but rather (even if unspoken), disgust. This tragic and inhumane instinctive misfire of the human brain fails to give individuals suffering from homelessness even a *chance* to be evaluated as a person. It blocks any appreciation for the real strength and beauty of resilience that is so often buried deep beneath the scars of their past. It also helps to explain how, when people who suffer from homelessness battle so hard to keep their heads above water, we can just look the other way and hold tight to our life preserver; how we routinely miss the opportunity to help, to love, and to live up to our preached ideals.

"The homeless" are labeled and disregarded, instantly and instinctively.

This study's findings clarified past experiences and revealed the root cause of so many hypocritical gaps between words and actions —gaps that political, social, and religious leaders over time had been trying to warn us about. Dr. Harris and Dr. Fiske's work helped identify the neurobiological mechanisms of these gaps—how entrenched and hardwired the instinct of judging and discarding "others" can be. Like so many other findings in their field, this helped to explain the mechanism underlying our human actions and predispositions throughout history.

From a homelessness perspective, the findings suggested that perhaps the main pathologies of chronic homelessness were societal rather than at the level of the individual experiencing homelessness. The issue was not necessarily about how the pathologies of those suffering from homelessness interact with the world, but rather how the world's pathologies interacted with them.

Seemingly, on the surface, these findings were pretty dark and hopeless. Thankfully, as we will come back to later, Dr. Harris dug deeper.

20

SOCIAL HIERARCHY

With an improved understanding of human social cognitive predispositions and their associated neuroanatomy comes a better insight into the challenges individuals encounter when they experience homelessness—the relentless barriers in their constant attempts to improve their social situations, as they work to navigate through complex, fragmented, and confusing collections of social and medical services.

Every social interaction is indeed two-sided. Each person brings their own strengths, weaknesses, and potential pathologies. The social activities of daily living—communication, social bonding, and more broadly, how we process and use information in social settings to direct behavior and interactions with others—primarily revolve around how we view ourselves relative to the person we're interacting with. When we meet somebody, we quickly judge where we should place them on a social hierarchy scale relative to ourselves. This helps direct the terms of the interaction, which makes a lot of sense from a social evolutionary perspective. It allows us to quickly prioritize our social efforts with those we're interacting with so we can, presumably, maximize our access to resources while optimizing our success—and therefore comfort—in a particular environment.

Those on top of the social hierarchy gain greater access to often-limited resources while frequently determining the flow of who gets what below them.

Research has demonstrated just how quickly these decisions around social hierarchy occur across species, including humans. A whole slew of subtle and likely subconsciously perceived social cues play into this, such as gaze, posturing, and tone. These all work to rapidly establish "asymmetrical displays of dominance," with relative positions of superiority or deference made and recognized within seconds.[1] The findings of Dr. Harris's study demonstrate just how automatic and anatomically hardwired this process can be.

The importance of such social ranking is evident in our daily lives.

From an early age, on the playgrounds and school hallways, we learn that people's perceptions of us help determine our rank in the societal hierarchies, which in turn dictate the terms of our daily social interactions. People spend a lot of time and effort optimizing their ranking—which causes a lot of insecurities, anxiety, and depression. This helps to explain "look at me" social media posts and people spending beyond their means on cars, homes, plastic surgery, and "$50 getting-tricked-by-a-business T-shirts" as advertisements of success aimed at improving social standing and hierarchy placement. All in an effort, presumably, to make life easier.

Studies have demonstrated some validity to this. It turns out we have different rules and expectations for people based on their social status rankings. People who are perceived as being higher on social hierarchies have been found to "get away with more"—waived speeding tickets, forgiveness for lying, shoulder shrugging for high-ranking politicians who don't experience the same consequences as everybody else. "Advantage begets advantage," and the uglier opposite end of that spectrum is also true.

As it turns out, those at the top need this leniency more. Research has demonstrated that individuals ranking higher in social status are often more likely to cheat, lie, break the law, and display unethical behavior if it's to their advantage to do so.[2] Yet, they are, ironically, more likely to be perceived as trustworthy.[3]

Social Hierarchy

We are intrinsically poor judges of character. When forming opinions or making judgments about others, we prioritize, often erroneously, our perception of their social hierarchy instead of our interpretations of their displayed personal attributes. The biblical warning about "judge not" seems to be right on; judge not, because instinctively we apparently suck at it.

Like so many neuroanatomical processes in our bodies, social cognition involves common pathways for the spectrum of social interactions we encounter, rather than a network of individualized ones for each social scenario. We don't have separate pathways for separate kinds of relationships. As Stanford neurobiologist, Dr. Andrew Huberman, states in his podcast on social bonding: "The neural circuits ... and the hormones ... are not unique to particular social bonds. They are generic—the same brain circuits that are responsible for establishing a bond between parents and child are actually repurposed in romantic relationships ...."[4]

For those who suffer from ACEs and their neuroanatomic impact, the ability to form strong social connections is often compromised early in life. Relationships based in trauma, abuse, and dehumanization rather than supportive love can alter the development of social connection pathways in the brain.

These neuroanatomical pathways related to social cognition form early in our lives. Children quickly learn and adapt to the structure of their social world, assigning rank within social structures and associating higher rank with more resources.[5] Children perceived to be athletic, good-looking, or wealthy receive praise and admiration from their peers, while others perceived to be lower on the social hierarchy are often bullied and teased. This can result in *Lord of the Flies*-type scenarios, as young kids try to put down others to improve their relative position, often almost instinctively.

Social stigmatization around homelessness also occurs at a young age—and when children are targeted by other children, it's often much more brutal and much less disguised than when this is done as adults. Mothers, fathers, and caregivers of children who suffer from homelessness are very aware of this, typically desperate to protect their children from potential bullying related to their social situations. Family shelters ensure children are picked up at a bus stop away from their buildings. They work hard to ensure kids have the necessary clothes and supplies to attend school. But even with these efforts, they often are unsuccessful.

During COVID-19's first winter of 2020 to 2021, when shelter access was limited or even shut down at times, a group of us from WakeMed scrambled to help staff a temporary "white flag" shelter on the nights when the weather was dangerously cold. Over a few weeks, I got to know an inspirational mother of two with a story of misfortunes that resulted in her living with her kids in her small sedan. When the weather would drop below freezing, and we would open the makeshift overnight shelter at a local church, she and her young son and daughter would come stay to protect themselves from the cold.

The mother was dynamic and articulate, with an engaging presence. There was something about how she maintained eye contact and asked questions, and just her overall social confidence, that defiantly challenged every existing stereotype that may have tried to force her down on social hierarchy scales. Her natural confidence and poise made the tragic consequences of her life resulting in homelessness seem that much more tragic.

Like many others at the white flag shelter, she struggled to sleep at night. She would walk to the lobby to hang out and talk with the skeleton volunteer staff who were trying to stay awake during the overnight shift. Later, as things became more settled and our initial skeleton crew evolved into a more structured environment with security and rules, this would end. But it was fun while it lasted.

People are often much more introspective during 2 a.m. conversations. Some amazingly insightful conversations occurred in the small lobby of the church-turned-shelter over the course of that winter.

This mother shared that her eight-year-old son, AJ, was being bullied relentlessly at school by a group of boys who had learned he and his family lived in their car. Her son was sweet, very quiet, and had an amazing, confident smile that lit up the room—which provided an inspirational irony to the darkness he was being forced to grow up in. Or perhaps it was a testament to the determined love of his mother who somehow maintained this light through this darkness. His classmates, the very first week of school that year, nicknamed him "Hobo." They teased him incessantly about any external manifestation of homelessness they could pick up on—old, worn-out shoes, hand-me-down clothes, poor hygiene. They made sure he suffered all the humiliations associated with the social situation he and his family were surviving, likely to boost their own insecurities as they fought for their own placement on the all-important grade-school social hierarchy scale.

At the overnight shelter, AJ watched his energetic younger sister with a love and patience that was inspirational. He had an extraordinary resilience, displayed by that smile and consistent physical posturing of standing straight—"never bowing his head"—which effectively seemed to not only insulate the blows but likely also to make them seem relatively weak and desperate. His mother believed the kids who bullied him even picked up on the fact that their attempts didn't seem to break him into submission. Or at least they saw that he was determined not to allow others' views to affect his self-perception and confidence (which is a tough thing to do). A few times, this resulted in him being physically assaulted.

"But they never broke him," she said, with both a tone of pride but also amazement. "They *never* broke him." One night, he came back from school with a bloody lip and a black eye. He said he tripped. That evening, he played Go Fish all night in the car with his little sister, "laughing the whole time with her as if nothing happened." Throughout all of this, he was able to maintain straight As in school.

If AJ isn't one day a CEO or in some sort of leadership position, it will be our society's loss. I pray the decks are not stacked too much against him, but as a young, Black child growing up homeless, they very well might be.

While exceptional and extraordinary, AJ's confidence and demeanor were unfair to expect as the norm.

Homelessness, ACEs, or merely social manifestations of extreme poverty all work to predispose children to reflexive demotion on the social hierarchies of the personal interactions that shape their lives. Incarcerated or "addicted" patients, hand-me-down clothes, and shelter addresses all work against gaining the respect, admiration, or even love of others—and themselves. The negative impact on self-perception and confidence is just one of ACEs' many damaging consequences. If a child gets told enough that they're low on the social hierarchy, especially if they're treated as such through the violence and dehumanization of ACEs, they're eventually going to believe it—even if they're a badass, resilient kid constantly fighting through challenges and adversity most of us can't relate to.

Society often forces these children on a trajectory early in their lives, and then penalizes and humiliates them for being on it as they age. Their incredible and inspirational resilience frequently goes unnoticed and unappreciated—by themselves and others.

When it comes to their daily interactions with others, which are often very few, people living on the streets or in homeless shelters are instinctively placed low down on social hierarchy scales by most people they interact with. They enter into almost every interaction with inflexible stereotypes, preconceptions, and labels designating them as "the lesser." Reflexive dehumanization is tough to overcome socially; to have to do it constantly is exhausting, frustrating, and potentially triggering. It often forces individuals into a defensive and potentially confrontational mode.

We've all had social confrontations when we feel disrespected or not listened to. They are stressful, especially as they escalate. You feel your heart rate increases. You might get flushed or start to sweat. As thoughts start to race, it can often feel like an out-of-body experience with parts of your brain shutting down. That is because, to some extent, parts of your brain *are*, in fact, shutting down. The flood of cortisol and adrenaline activating these stress-related responses in your body prioritizes activity in the reactive part of the brain—the amygdala and other parts of the limbic system—while shutting down those associated with cognition, compassion, or problem-solving. We stop communicating and thinking. Instead, we start reacting.

You may have worked to recognize this when it happens—whether in your work, family, or social life—and come up with coping mechanisms and strategies. You may have applied your own versions of "mindfulness"—trying to breathe, relax, bring down your pulse, and rationalize the situation to put into perspective that it doesn't warrant getting this worked up over.

Yet, it can be challenging. Calming down an emotionally reacting brain is easier said than done. This is especially true in individuals who suffer from historical trauma and its neuroanatomic complications of ramped-up, trigger-able, and hypertrophied, reactive neurologic systems—making it extra hard to navigate perceived threats and conflict resolution.

People who suffer from homelessness are often forced to have most social interactions in this reactive mindset. They are put on the defensive through reflexive dehumanization. From a neuroanatomic perspective, they have both hands tied behind their back as they engage with others in the world around them. Socializing can almost become an impossible task—typically, one they are given very little time to perform. Instead, their social interactions are typically brief and often dismissive—without time to make connections or even to convey their humanity.

If most of a person's social interactions are unpleasant, this can, over time, result in progressively worsening social isolation. People would often rather live alone than have to expose themselves to the constant social trauma of dehumanization.

Our brain works just as hard to avoid negative social interactions as it does to seek out positive ones. Over time, with primarily negative patterns of social interactions, this will result in a "social homeostasis," driven by the basal lateral aspect of the amygdala[6] that predisposes someone to seek isolation. The experience of trauma itself can predispose an overactive and hypertrophied amygdala to avoid, or at least minimize, exposure to painful, toxic social interactions.

As homelessness and its associated isolation become more chronic, I've seen my patients increasingly withdraw from society. Loneliness shares a common trait of so many of the great human diseases; its symptoms circle back to worsen its underlying pathology. Loneliness results in more loneliness, which snowballs into increased social dysfunction.

This not only leads to stress, sadness, and decreased quality of life, but also to crappy neurotransmitter balances, illness, and early deaths.

21

LONELINESS

The most terrible poverty is loneliness,
and the feeling of being unloved.
—Mother Teresa

A few years back, I gained an interest—an expertise really, at least according to me—in telling hilarious dad jokes. One day in clinic, I shared a hilarious one with the staff:

"What did the fish say when he hit the wall?"

"Dam!"

All morning, my staff resisted admitting it was hilarious. One of my patients overheard our conversations as he was being weighed and roomed in the clinic.

He was a new patient, John, who had come in that day for evaluation for his diabetes. He had just come to Raleigh and had been chronically homeless for years. He was in his 50s, with leathery, tanned skin from the constant sun exposure while living outside. Soft-spoken, he had a persistent "smile in his eyes." He also had a quickly evident and striking wisdom about him. I was instantly intrigued by him but rapidly distracted by the question he tossed my way before I could sit down: "So what was the joke?"

This was really all I needed; he'd opened the door a crack, so I busted through and shared the joke with him. He laughed. Really laughed—not an obligatory or apologetic laugh, but a legitimate one. After he was done, he looked up, and with much more introspection than a cheesy dad joke seemed to warrant, stated: "You know, that was the first time somebody has told me a joke in years. Got to remember that one." He seemed surprised, nostalgic, and even sad as he reflected on this.

His story, when we got into it, was both fascinating and also intentionally mysterious. He wasn't too interested in sharing his pain or complaining about anything; he just wanted his A1C (test of diabetic control) and blood pressure checked. But he did share that he had been homeless for "years and years" and was very nomadic, constantly traveling from city to city. He had crossed back and forth across our nation several times over, only staying at each location for a few months. This was his first time in North Carolina.

"Got to keep moving," he said when I asked him about this pattern.

"Why is that?" I replied.

"So much to see," he responded in what seemed like a guarded attempt to hide the real answers he didn't want to reveal.

As he left (his blood pressure and A1C both looked great), I felt like I probably wouldn't see him again. I was right.

At lunch that day, the front desk brought me a folded piece of paper sealed with scotch tape. Before he left, I'd handed John a diabetic educational handout on diet and exercise, which he initially had refused, saying, "I've heard it all before." However, it was so well written I pushed for him to at least take it and see if there was anything new he could learn from it.

I opened the folded piece of paper to find this handout (I couldn't help but feel like there was a passive-aggressive, middle-fingerish-type message in there). On the back of the handout, he'd scribbled a few sentences in somewhat tremulous, relatively sloppy writing. He seemed to be putting into words questions he'd been unable to articulate when we spoke: *Where can I find happiness? What if no one cares? Where do I go?* Curiously, he signed the note "CS"—not his own initials—and then next to that scribbled the word *Roadsinger*. That was it. Nothing more.

I did not recognize the words but wondered if they had a deeper meaning. I did what anybody does when they don't know something nowadays: I googled it. I discovered that John's message seemed to be trying to reference the song "Roadsinger," written by Yusuf Islam (formerly known by his stage name, Cat Stevens) in 2012.

I was surprised he took the time to write this before leaving. It seemed vulnerable from someone who was so guarded.

The whole interaction was a bit surreal—but so are many interactions with our patients. I wish I'd had the opportunity to know John better. I got the sense that he held on to a lot of important insights from his experiences that would have been fascinating to see if I could have wrangled them out of him. I also got the sense, however, that he really had no interest in sharing them.

It's a hundred little things coming to us in our daily interactions with our environments and other people that make us human and provide meaning in life.

Missing these little things can be what hurts the most.

When you're homeless, it can be difficult to truly appreciate just how much has been taken from you. Little glimpses of the love, laughter, and good in life—which can occasionally burst through the darkness—can contain nostalgic reminders of better days. Those days still may have been filled with trauma and pain, but perhaps contained more hope—and relationships.

For the most part, many people experiencing chronic homelessness can spend their lives in isolation. They'll often go days without anybody calling them by their name. Or greeting them. They'll often go months without people laughing with them, crying with them, or showing them validation or support. Instead, and in contrast to most of our lives, they go unnoticed. Or if they are noticed, it is with scorn, stereotypes, and judgments—on the streets, in the hospitals, or in shelters.

Loneliness is the greatest pain of homelessness. It can also be one of its most damaging health consequences.

Human beings have evolved as a social species. We need and

crave interactions with others. Studies have demonstrated that our relationships with others are the primary determinants of our happiness—and health.

Harvard psychiatrist Dr. Robert Waldinger gave a TED talk in 2015 about his research on determinants of happiness. As part of an extraordinary longitudinal study that started tracking 238 Harvard sophomores in 1938 and followed them throughout their lifetime, his team has identified that relationships are far more important to happiness than financial success or fame/reputation. *Close* relationships. Dr. Waldinger explained: "The clearest message that we get from this 75-year study is this: Good relationships keep us happier and healthier, period. We've learned ... that social connections are really good for us and that loneliness kills. It turns out that people who are more socially connected to family, to friends, to community are happier, they are physically healthier and they live longer than people who are less well connected. And the experience of loneliness turns out to be toxic. People who are more isolated than they want to be from others find that they are less happy, their health declines earlier in midlife, their brain functioning declines sooner and they live shorter lives."[1]

In 2023, the Surgeon General released an advisory warning that provided more insights into these harmful impacts of loneliness on our social, mental, and physical health. The report cited: "The physical health consequences of poor or insufficient connection include a 29 percent increased risk of heart disease, a 32 percent increased risk of stroke, and a 50 percent increased risk of developing dementia for older adults. Additionally, lacking social connection increases risk of premature death by more than 60 percent."[2] This equates to the health equivalent of smoking 15 cigarettes per day.[3]

Mother Theresa was right: The most terrible poverty, and likely one of our greatest health risk factors, is loneliness—the feeling of being unloved. Over time, it crushes happiness, health, and eventually hope. In my experience, it is the loss of hope that can be the loudest death knell of homelessness.

22

TWENTY-SEVEN POUNDS OF CHAINS

The majority of women who experience chronic homelessness have experienced a brutal form of trauma that has been proven to drive its victims into social isolation.

During the COVID Omicron surge in the winter of 2021 to 2022, more than a year and a half into the pandemic, we still hadn't figured it all out and were scrambling yet again to manage another wave of infections. As cases spread like wildfire in our local homeless community, those not sick enough to require hospitalization needed a place to recover, as hospital bed access was becoming dangerously low. The shelters, under quarantine and restrictions, had limited capacity. So we partnered with a local hotel, set up one of their rooms as our office, and tried to do our best. We were anticipating managing perhaps 5 to 10 patients at a time at the hotel. By early January 2022, our census was over 50. We would eventually serve more than 230 COVID-positive patients with housing insecurities in this hotel.

In the middle of the surge, I received a call from Detective Wendy Clark who helped to run the Raleigh Police Department's Addressing Crises through Outreach, Referrals, Networking, and Service (ACORNS) team. She was concerned about an elderly female who lived on the streets and had tested positive for COVID the day before at a local community clinic. With cold weather coming, this woman was starting to feel sick. Detective Clark called to inquire about the hotel.

At that time, it was hard to ask anybody to transport COVID-positive patients in their car—and we couldn't really advise them to use public transportation (would be poor form). So the path of least resistance was often my super cool 2015 Honda Pilot.

I drove downtown and met her at Raleigh's Moore Square.

As we were getting her into the car, she struggled to raise her legs. We had to assist, helping her to get each leg into the car, one at a time. The reason: She wore 27 pounds of metal chains, with multiple locks, around her waist. (These would be weighed a few months later, after she agreed—following successful case management engagement and improvement in her mental health—to have the chains removed, so she could get a necessary CT scan during an emergency room visit.) She had been the victim of multiple past sexual assaults. This was her solution. Out of necessity and desperation. She spent her days walking the streets—in her 60s, suffering from arthritis and lung disease—with a 27-pound "chastity belt," as she called it.

There is no greater, or more obvious, form of dehumanization than the objectification of women and associated acts of trauma and violence.

If you read enough statistics, your mind can become numb to the very reality they shine a light on.

In a study of a large, racially diverse sample of homeless mothers in 1997, 92 percent had experienced severe physical and/or sexual abuse at some point in their lives[1]… 92 percent!

In a study we performed at a resident program that served homeless women suffering from addiction, 58 percent of participants reported being victims of sexual abuse as children.

In another study, 13 percent of a sample of homeless women reported having been raped in the past 12 months, and half of these women were raped at least twice.[2] In homeless youth, 61 percent of girls and 16 percent of boys report sexual abuse at home as a reason for running away.[3] One in three teens will be recruited by a pimp within 48 hours of leaving home.[4]

We see similar patterns of violence in transgender populations, with a 2022 study of approximately 1,000 participants demonstrating that 47 percent had been sexually assaulted in their lives, with approximately 20 percent at one time having experienced homelessness.[5]

There are many disturbing statistics around the pain, suffering, and root cause of homelessness. There are likely none more troubling than these.

Horrific, violent acts of dehumanization early in life often force their victims onto firm trajectories toward suffering ... and isolation, as studies have demonstrated that victims of sexual abuse are more likely to withdraw into the damaging outcomes of social isolation discussed by Dr. Waldinger and highlighted in the Surgeon General's warning.[6,7]

Addiction often provides relief. Pathology builds on pathology. Abuse circles back to pave the way for future trauma, which contributes to expensive suffering, early deaths, and 27-pound chastity belts worn out of desperation.

Yet we have very much struggled to adequately address historic trauma in our populations experiencing homelessness. Women who suffer from homelessness are often still openly sexually harassed or even abused in public. Staff members at homeless shelters and in medical communities are often not appropriately trained on how to screen for, and respond appropriately to, sexual violence and trauma. The stigmatization of homelessness itself presents barriers when women try to address reported harassment with law enforcement or social and medical services. While the #MeToo movement has placed an increased spotlight on sexual abuse and harassment nationally, people often aren't listening to homeless women; and so they continue to suffer alone, in social isolation with all its deadly consequences.

23

THE BEAM

The interactions that occur in medical settings are simply a microcosm of our larger society.

Physicians and other healthcare employees, typically well-respected and well-compensated, have historically been at the top of their social hierarchies, especially in America. This includes in the daily provider-patient interactions that serve as the foundation of medicine.

These interactions occur on medicine's terms. Medical providers typically assume the role of dominance atop the hierarchy, as they have the particular abilities needed to run their environment to the perceived benefit of all in it. This inevitably creates an uneven playing field for those patients seeking care who may have to advocate for themselves—especially if they are reflexively perceived as being far down on the social hierarchy scale.

Historically, medical providers' interactions with their patients have often involved more orders and instructions than two-way conversations. Empowering patients with knowledge about their health and conditions has never been a major priority. For the most part, we as providers have driven the decisions. All of which may be more acceptable if not for that fact that one-third of everything we have ordered and instructed has been futile,[1] or the fact that an estimated 250,000 Americans die per year due to medical errors.[2] Most people who have been in a medical environment realize there is often a need for self-advocacy as they interact with the expensive churnings of our massive healthcare system. Often, family members will assist as important advocates for loved ones.

There's nothing more frustrating as a patient, especially a sick patient, than the feeling they're not being listened to. Poor provider communication is a driver of not only poor patient satisfaction but also patient adherence to treatment plans and, therefore, actual medical outcomes.[3] If we hope to gain the trust and engagement of our patients to maximize health outcomes and therefore our success as providers, our patients must believe that our interactions with them are genuine—unbiased and unselfish, with their best interest in mind. The patient must feel like they're seen as equal, or even "superior" partners on any social hierarchy for our particular interactions. They must feel like they're part of the conversation. They cannot sense an arrogant entitlement of superiority, and definitely not a sense of disgust. Patients, especially those who have a lot of experience with it, can recognize when they're not being listened to —seeing through superficial "bless-your-hearts" and disingenuous attempts at compassion. They can (very easily) tell when they're being pushed down on the social hierarchy scale and treated as incompetent or unintelligent.

Gaining patient trust is absolutely a prerequisite to clinical success, especially in historically marginalized populations. We've just been really bad at our strategies for obtaining it. If we're successful, however, trust can be leveraged into longer-term clinical relationships and associated improved outcomes.

Our job in medicine is simple: Work with patients to alleviate suffering to the best of our abilities by treating—or even better in value-based models, *preventing*—disease. In doing so, we aim to increase both their quality and quantity of life.

We trained for years to learn how to best do this. It starts with well-informed knowledge of the pathologies that harm our patients, so we can identify them when present (diagnosis). We then treat. We were trained and now get paid to think through the treatment process. To use our cognitive and executive function capabilities to solve very complex problems. To understand pathology so as to better address and treat it. We do not get paid to simply assert social hierarchy dominance, or to get frustrated by, or worse, reflexively blame patients for, the pathologies they're suffering from.

Yet, this is what we do on a daily basis when patients come into our medical silos.

We hate defeat or the demonstrations of our ignorance in the poor outcomes of our patients. Blaming patients is a defense mechanism used to protect our egos in medicine, which admittedly are relatively large. We use the tools of labels, stereotypes, and bias to accomplish this as we blame patients for the challenging manifestations of mental health and trauma that we don't know how to effectively treat.

Words matter. Societal labels based on stereotypes are a primary weapon used to quickly facilitate the reflexive dehumanization Dr. Harris identified in his functional MRIs. Society uses a variety of labels: "bums," "addicts," "beggars," "vagrants"—to strip individuals experiencing homelessness of their humanity, reducing them to just a single aspect of their identity. These are meant to help delegate a person to a preconceived and typically negative assessment without affording them the chance of being socially evaluated and judged as an individual or an equal.

As we discussed earlier, whatever mission statement or religious or social ideals you follow, a foundational aspect to most is *love*—or at least enough respect to evaluate each person for who they actually are. This is a basic prerequisite to any logical and efficient human interaction, and the failure to do so is the fault of the dismisser.

The goal of labels and stereotypes is always selfish. They are lazy and dangerous filters in our social interactions—judgmental shortcuts that quickly assign social hierarchy ranking to people we interact with. They save us time and energy by not requiring us to personally assess an individual, instead allowing us to bypass straight to the desired outcome—with us on top and the person we are labeling typically placed below us.

By definition, most labels imply a relative sense of worthlessness by conjuring up common and historical stereotypes. Over time, this has been expanded to the very illnesses we misunderstood and mismanaged being used as the labels themselves—an *addict*, or *schizophrenic*, or *histrionic*. Such diagnoses can trigger a reflexive bias that results in a different level of conversation, listening, diagnosis, and care.

In medicine, one of the most dangerous, expensive, but common labels we see is "malingering." This is a diagnosis given by a health provider when they believe a patient is presenting more for secondary gain—to get something—than for medical reasons. Admittedly, hospitals in any community serve as the ultimate safety net for their residents. When a person has nowhere else to turn and feels their safety and health are in danger, they can always come to the hospital. Unlike social service agencies, churches, or other organizations, hospitals are open 24 hours a day, never closing.

Crushing chest pain, unable to speak, struggling to breathe, a desperate sense of hopelessness, thinking about killing themselves, drowning in addiction, feeling like they have no other safe options—people fall into our hospitals' safety nets for a number of complex reasons. For those who suffer from homelessness, who often live in isolation without other supporting social safety nets, they will frequently come to us when they don't perceive having a safer option in their often brutal daily struggle to survive. This is especially true in patients with mental illness.

Malingering is very much an overused and misunderstood diagnosis in medicine that we often see in the charts of those experiencing homelessness.

When used, the provider basically concludes that the patient is "consciously simulating" whatever symptoms they're presenting with for "secondary gain."

It should always be a diagnosis of exclusion.

Once the diagnosis is in a patient's chart, it follows them; they are labeled in a way that can bias their care and affect medical decisions. A "malingerer" who presents with medical complaints will often be ignored and their conditions not believed but quickly discarded as fabricated.

It has dangerous implications around bias as well. The term malingering was found to be used twice as much in the inpatient setting with Black patients compared to the general population.[4]

In times of stress on health systems, such as during COVID or bed shortages, we see utilization of this label increase. I don't think it's a coincidence, as providers under stress are more apt to give into bias and the convenience it provides.

Early in my career, I had a patient who went to a local ER complaining he was tired of being homeless. Tired of being cold during a brutal winter. He felt like he wanted to end his life, as he couldn't take it anymore. He planned to walk out in traffic. The ER notes referenced and acknowledged this, but it was concluded that he didn't need admission, as it was believed he was "exaggerating" his symptoms. On his discharge note, he was given the diagnosis of malingering. Four days later, he returned to the ER, brought in by ambulance after being hit by a car. He was dead on arrival.

It's hard to exaggerate the pain of homelessness. If people seem miserable, it's usually because they are. If we pause and listen, it's usually not hard to tell why. If we listen better, we might be able to act earlier to avoid the poor outcomes that contribute to a life expectancy that is 20-plus years below the national average, and financial costs that dwarf those of non-homeless populations.

Admittedly, it's incredibly hard not to fall into the trap of reaction and subsequent blame, as moving away from it requires medical providers to both recognize and then push back against so many of our *own* social instincts.

But, many things are incredibly hard in medicine. Curing different types of cancer, finding an effective HIV or hepatitis C treatment, developing the technology to do minimally invasive robotic surgery to improve patient outcomes. All of these things were incredibly hard to do. Forty years ago, everything listed above would have been perceived as impossible. But medicine is at its best when it's challenged with the difficult. Through research, experience, and the incredible innovation and determination that is the foundation of American medicine, we've made progress in improving patient outcomes.

However, we haven't been as determined and innovative when it comes to problem-solving in settings outside of the controlled environments of our labs and clinics—in how we approach social interactions, patient engagement, or behavioral modification. While American medicine has continued to lead the rest of the world in terms of impressive (and expensive) technology and therapies, we have failed to advance in the much "simpler" and basic goals of improving patient engagement and trust. Once again, this is especially true in populations that have been historically marginalized into health inequities and disparities.

The reality is that it's *not* all that simple. It is complex and often involves the neurobiology and social pathologies of human behavior in both patients *and* us as providers. It can also involve conceding control and our positions atop social hierarchies. It is hard to change our mindsets. But if we apply the same level of determination and innovation as we do in other fields of medicine to improve, the potential impact on patient outcomes and associated cost can be tremendous.

24

THE FOUR RS

Within a decade of President Garfield's death due to germ-theory ignorance, doctors were routinely washing their hands. They had a better understanding of pathology and its underlying mechanisms, and adjusted accordingly to improve patient outcomes.

Similarly, systems across the country are starting to appreciate the clinical importance of becoming "trauma-informed" to help improve the efficiency (and the humanity) of their patient care by better addressing both patient and medical provider pathologies. Honestly, when most medical providers and staff hear about this, especially in today's enlightened-buzzword environment, the immediate response is often skepticism and exhaustion. It's reflexively misinterpreted as some trendy "ideal of the month" initiative instead of what it is: a clinical strategy that will result in better and more efficient outcomes—and make our jobs as clinicians easier. This can be especially true with the highest risk, often most expensive patients who are becoming increasingly important to manage efficiently for those medical systems seeking to evolve toward value models that hold them accountable for cost and performance.

As my colleagues, Dr. Jaclyn Fremont, Dr. Pascal Udekwu, and I wrote in an opinion piece in *JAMA Surgery* on the topic: "Said plainly, trauma-informed care acknowledges that a person's health and well-being are the results of individual life experiences, environmental and societal stressors, and the institutional power structure. To be trauma informed, we ... must recognize these determinants in patients, and, as a healthcare system, we must be able to integrate a patient's past trauma into current and future care. For example, rather than blaming patients out of frustration for the pathologies they evince and demanding 'what is wrong with this patient?' we should instead ask 'what happened to them?' and 'how can I help?'"[1]

That's our role. To help. Not to blame. To problem-solve in an effort to help. Period—no more, no less.

Different levels of training exist around trauma-informed care, many of which can become overly complicated and therefore miss the main, digestible, and memorable takeaways. I personally like the "Four R" approach as a first step. Applied not only in medicine but also in schools and across different community and social service sectors, it guides staff in their daily interactions with those who may suffer from historic trauma.

(Please indulge me here for the next two pages as I present the very basics of this approach, as I truly believe if we can all learn the basics of this—inside and outside of medicine—we can be a much cooler and friendlier society.)

The first R: *Realize* what trauma is and how it can impact people and your interaction with them. This goes back to the basic idea that *knowledge of mechanism is everything*. What is the science and pathophysiology of trauma? We can't recognize that with which we're unfamiliar. The neurobiology and physiological impact of chronic trauma and stress—and its impact on the brain and medical outcomes—should be a foundational part of medical training, just like diabetes or the Krebs cycle (especially the Krebs cycle!). It's safe to say that most providers currently know very little, if anything, about the impact of trauma on the physiology and medical outcomes of the patients they serve. What are the stressors people face in their daily lives—poverty, abuse, toxic neighborhood environments, racism—and how do they impact their health and interactions with medical providers? Chronic toxic stress is one of the most common, damaging, expensive, and overlooked pathologies we see in medicine. If we know what it is, we can be on the lookout for it ... which leads to the second R.

The second R: *Recognize* the signs of trauma when we see it. Again, like diabetes or any disease, once we have an understanding of what trauma is, we can learn how to recognize it when we see it. Basically, this is *diagnosis*: knowing what we're dealing with, so we can treat it. When we successfully recognize trauma and its symptoms, we can cognitively think to address it instead of reflexively reacting to exacerbate it. For me, I've learned the earlier I can do this in patient interactions, the better. If I can recognize and adjust to it rather than getting frustrated by it, I can go into a clinical problem-solving mode to hopefully minimize its impact and my potential to exacerbate it. Knowing this makes my job of treating the patient much, much easier—and more rewarding.

The third R: *Respond* to trauma, when recognized, with established processes and workflows. This focus must be on a system level. The entire experience of interacting with medical providers, ER rooms, and hospitals can be traumatizing and retriggering for patients. The patient experience starts when they walk through the door and continues until they leave. Providers are often only a relatively small part of a patient's clinical experience. Anybody who has worked in clinical practice knows of the importance of good front desk staff, medical assistants, and nursing. The tone of the visit is often set by the patients' interactions with clinic staff well before we even walk into the room. To address trauma effectively, you need an informed model across the system with buy-in from all staff.

The fourth R: *Resist re-traumatization*. A foundational component of the Hippocratic Oath, as I've mentioned, is "do no harm." Given what we know about the biological responses when people are thrown back into a traumatizing or stressful situation, the horse can get out of the barn early on both sides of the patient-provider equation, resulting in further harm. Once out, it's hard to get that horse back in. When we see somebody go into a confrontational or fight mode, for example, we naturally do the same in response. Our frustration around the patient's reactivity leads to our own, and the snowball of dysfunction starts to roll and grow. Two battling amygdalae rarely result in effective social interactions—including in medicine.[2]

In my career, working through this process of becoming trauma-informed has been a clinical game-changer. It has converted any worsening burnout after 15 years of practicing homeless medicine into improved understanding, fascination, hope, and ultimately, improved patient outcomes.

As with most providers, I assume most of my patient interactions will be easy from a social perspective—friendly, rewarding, and without conflict. On a clinical day, the interactions with 19 out of the 20 patients on a provider's schedule can be excellent, but all it takes is one to throw them off their clinical game—to frustrate them. The same is true for our daily social interactions. One poor social interaction can ruin a day of otherwise positive ones.

Confrontational or angry interactions can knock medical providers off their social and cognitive flow for the day. We're gaining a better appreciation for why this is. For one, it blocks the very prefrontal lobe executive function we need to do our job. There's no greater time-suck in medicine, or really in life, than engaging in avoidable conflict. Frustration and arguments are time-consuming and typically not productive. They aren't billable. They rarely improve outcomes. They destroy patient comfort and satisfaction. Conflict is usually pointless, and when you really think about it, almost always avoidable.

The biggest argument for trauma-informed care is that it's a clinical strategy that can make our lives easier as providers, not harder. Forget compassion (if you want to); the argument becomes about increased efficiency in the job we're paid to do.

To be able to recognize the signs and symptoms of conflict and understand their root cause—to switch that conversation from, "What's wrong with this patient?" to, "How can I help?"—can add perspective to these interactions in real-time and turn them into fascinating cognitive challenges instead of emotional or personal threats. Practicing a sort of "clinical mindfulness" at the point of care, before the adrenaline horse gets out of the barn on both sides, allows us as providers to remain efficiently inside of our thinking, problem-solving mode, instead of slipping into a reactive one. This is an incredible clinical strategy. It flips frustration into motivation and irritation into sympathy. In many cases, it can turn failure into success.

Our goal in medicine should not be to get selfish dopamine hits from displays of social superiority or our own personal validation. It should be to treat the pathology in front of us that is resulting in our patient's suffering. Let the patient be heard and understood, and allow *them* the therapeutic dopamine hits. They likely need it more than we do.

Proactively addressing trauma rather than reacting to it can feel really challenging, and to avoid sounding sanctimonious, after all these years, I still constantly struggle with it. But it's possible—and necessary. Fortunately, I have some incredible examples in my life of people who mastered the art of making it look easy.

25

LISTEN

Blu Honeycutt was never a patient of mine. But she will always be one of my role models.

COVID hit our nation's homeless communities with a vengeance. In March 2020, we saw the storm coming. Our medical team worked feverishly to help prepare for a pandemic we knew would inevitably impact the homeless community more than the rest of society.

In medicine, we use data, studies, and experiences over years to help develop guidelines and treatment protocols. At the time, just months into the COVID pandemic, we were flying blind, scrambling to piece together the little information available to determine the best approach.

Our homeless community had questions like the rest of us, but with less access to answers.

Since 2016, we had been operating a "patient grand round lecture series" for the guests of local homeless shelters and programs, eventually held at Oak City Cares. This is an incredible facility built in 2019 that serves as a central hub for coordinated services and programs to assist those who are at risk of, or experiencing, homelessness.

The lecture series was an adaption of the historic "grand rounds" educational lectures that are typically held in hospital and academic settings. They involve medical providers learning from experts who are presenting in their particular medical specialty. These educational opportunities help keep health professionals up-to-date on the latest medical developments. We flipped the idea to focus on patient health education—empowering participants through knowledge to make informed health decisions and improve their health in the context of the unique challenges posed by homelessness.

On Wednesdays, we regularly transformed the large dining room at Oak City Cares into a makeshift classroom for our lunchtime lectures. Over a meal (typically pizza and salad—arguably not the healthiest option for our guests but unarguably delicious and well appreciated)—we would have conversations about health topics of interest to the community. No matter the topic of the particular lecture—mental health, preventive health, trauma, the opioid epidemic, heart disease, cold/heat exposure—the talks were always interesting to give. They were so successful, and felt so important, that we expanded the lecture series into a true community collaboration, with guest speakers from Duke, UNC, and the county health department. Participants had incredible questions and insights. I was often left thinking how nice it would be if the students and residents I taught were half as engaged as the guests at these lectures.

In early March 2020, we started to plan for a lecture on COVID to provide information and guidance to the Oak City Cares guests. However, as the pandemic started to quickly spread in our community, it became clear we were running out of time.

We knew we were soon going to lose the ability to bring people together to provide education. We were about to become socially isolated. We knew we must act quickly.

On the morning of March 6, I hopped on a call with Oak City staff. A few hours later, we were in the large dining hall, eating pizza and working to explain COVID the best we could: Try not to touch your face. Wash your hands. Wear masks ... or do not wear masks (we were still uncertain at the time, and the rush on masks in the general population ensured there were virtually none left for our guests). Several people asked questions about conspiracy theories, even that early.

The lectures were usually fun, engaging, and awesome. The March 6, 2020, lecture was the opposite. People were scared, hesitant, and confused. I did little to help. I usually left the grand round lectures feeling inspired. That day, I left feeling nervous and clueless.

The situation was all new and evolving quickly. As I would continue to do throughout the COVID-19 pandemic, I referenced the most updated Centers for Disease Control and Prevention (CDC) and state health department guidelines the best I could. However, these recommendations failed early on in the pandemic to provide adequate guidance for patients facing the unique barriers associated with homelessness. As society was becoming familiar with recommendations around handwashing, mask-wearing, social distancing, and shelter-in-place orders, people without homes or shelter had no idea what to do. The whole thing felt a bit detached from reality. While we had an obligation to get out and let them know the storm was coming, we also couldn't offer any good advice as to what they could actually do to protect themselves. This clearly exposed—to them and to us—just how isolated they were. It was hard to hide the fact that, in all the early societal panic and reaction to COVID, those without housing were largely forgotten. Shelters were limiting access, programs were shutting down, and people were being forced to live outside without resources.

"What are we supposed to do?"

This simple, direct question was asked repeatedly. The half-assed answers around "do the best you can ... good luck" that paralleled those I threw out during the March 6 lecture were clearly insufficient. This was especially true for the sick and elderly in the population who were being forced to the street without support. They knew that. I knew that. Everybody knew that.

As a community, we spend so much time trying to address—and

if that's not possible, hide—the holes in our social safety nets that when we can't, it disturbingly rips down the fragile frameworks of justification and rationalization we often use to keep moving. COVID destroyed these frameworks, leaving us exposed and deflated.

Weeks later, fears played out across the nation for those suffering from homelessness. As our society shut down in social isolation, "the homeless" were often quickly forgotten by communities just trying to weather the storm. As most of us were mourning the closings of restaurants, businesses, and movie theaters, people suffering from homelessness were scrambling to survive the closings of life-sustaining assistance programs, street outreach teams, and shelter beds. As we all went running for cover, a familiar sense of abandonment was felt by those who were homeless. They had no cover.

Locally in Raleigh, we did the best we could—leveraging the unique level of collaboration in our community between local governments, nonprofit organizations, healthcare systems, and faith organizations. And while we fared better than most communities, especially with early and innovative efforts by the county to move the sick and elderly into hotel rooms, in the end, it wasn't nearly enough. Shelters and programs still had to reduce capacity. People were still left outside, which got increasingly dangerous as we headed into winter. As a community, like others around the nation, we were unable to provide basic shelter options for those suffering from homelessness. Addiction services and drop-in centers were also limited, compromising our ability to manage the mental health and addiction surges that accompanied COVID.

The eye of the storm with COVID, predictably, was a direct hit on the homeless population.

Mister Rogers, the children's television TV host, in all his happy, singing, suede-sweater awesomeness, had a great quote that is frequently referenced during challenging times: "When I was a boy and I would see scary things in the news, my mother would say to me, 'Look for the helpers. You will always find people who are helping.'"

As the storm of COVID hit, you didn't have to look hard to find Blu Honeycutt running into the middle of it, just as most were running in the opposite direction.

With her trademark blue hair, block-letter tattoos on her arm, and fatigueless smile, Blu was a peer support specialist who helped to operate Love Wins, a drop-in day shelter. This was one of the only sites that stayed open and fully functional during the pandemic, serving the increasing number of unhoused individuals forced to stay outside, with the shelters at limited capacity. It provided a place to eat, laugh, use the bathrooms, and shower. A large grass area outside allowed people to gather and talk, which was especially beneficial in trying to maintain safe social distancing practices to the extent possible. On nice days, when this grass area was full of people, it provided an almost festive contrast to the social isolation in the rest of society.

Love Wins provided a place to connect with their unsheltered guests, checking in on their health and sharing information. We used the location as part of our local effort to get elderly and sick homeless residents off the streets and into county-funded hotel rooms—such as a 73-year-old with advanced emphysema and a history of lung cancer who Blu contacted me about early in the pandemic. Blu was out there, every day, serving her unhoused friends who had nowhere else to go—smiling while fielding questions and requests for help from those who needed it.

One afternoon, I dropped off a box of 100 masks that we had managed to secure for Love Wins guests (which, at the time in May of 2020, felt like the greatest public health accomplishment of all time). I found Blu in the corner of the lawn, listening to a crying, disheveled woman. She excused herself to grab the masks.

"How are you doing?" I asked Blu.

"Hanging in there," she answered.

"Are you exhausted?"

This was more of a rhetorical question, as we were approaching two months into the pandemic. Not only was everybody exhausted, but it seemed everybody in society was telling everybody else just how exhausted they were—as part of a culturally accepted "group therapy" vibe.

"Hell no!" she said with a smile. And with a small laugh, she promptly returned to listening intently to the crying woman.

Blu continued her work as COVID progressed, developing street outreach teams with her friend Thomas to deliver food to homeless encampment sites. She was instrumental in our vaccination efforts once our patients experiencing homelessness (finally) became eligible. Our success rate with getting patients to agree to the vaccination would more than double if Blu was alongside us as we answered questions, filled out forms, and administered vaccines. If we wanted to engage a patient with particularly challenging mental health issues, we would often go through Blu and leverage the uniquely trusting relationships she'd worked to build with so many of our community's residents.

Blu mastered the art of listening. I was fascinated to see her interactions with others—how she leveraged listening into understanding, and then understanding into therapy and help. She made it look easy, and she would argue that was because it *was* easy. Her greatest skill was almost impossible to emulate: She listened *with joy*, as if she was genuinely appreciative of the honor of having somebody talk to her, share their story, and confide in her. She was always fully present, fully engaged, and locked in on the person she was talking to. Nothing offers a person more dignity than being truly listened to.

A few months before the pandemic hit, Blu was part of a talk on homelessness we gave in the community. She spoke about her life, her own experiences with homelessness, and her approach in working to help others. A guest captured her speech in a video he sent me a few months later, in which Blu explained: "When you walk by somebody and you just keep going, that is dehumanizing whether you realize it or not, because now you haven't stopped to say, 'Hey, this is who I am, and I am sorry you are in this situation. I don't have anything to give you, but I have a heart and I have ears; do you want to talk for a minute?' That means so much more than anything monetarily you can give somebody. *Re*-humanizing them is a big deal."

This was a message she would repeatedly emphasize and exemplify in her own life. It was simple: Listen.

Just stop ... and listen.

She implored us to try, because she knew if we did, our effort would almost always be successful. She knew it would routinely lead us to humanize one another, allowing us to avoid the reflexive traps of convenient stereotypes. Reflexive humanization is infinitely better than reflexive judging. She didn't know, and I imagine wouldn't really care, about Dr. Harris and Dr. Fiske's research that helps to explain the science and neuroanatomy supporting her message.

There was another fascinating, and perhaps optimistic, MRI finding in Dr. Harris and Dr. Fiske's study with those Princeton undergrad students. As the prefrontal cortex failed to trigger and humanize, and the anterior insula lit up in "disgust," they saw activity in another part of the brain: the anterior cingulate cortex. A collar-shaped region in the front part of the brain, it is responsible for many higher-level functions such as decision-making, morality, attention, and in the part that consistently lit up in Dr. Harris's study, conflict resolution. As the participants were reflexively dehumanizing, their brains were instinctively working to resolve the potential conflict in doing so. This led Dr. Harris and Dr. Fiske to hypothesize that "estimations of less typical humanity to social targets relate to increased conflict resolution, perhaps because participants are obviously aware that the targets are indeed human beings."[1]

As Dr. Harris would later explain: "We have developed this as a strategy to get us through our social environment. Most people think, and rightly so, that homeless people are having very negative experiences and constantly suffering. We may not always want to resonate with that suffering."[2] So our brains alter and censor these perceptions to prevent unpleasant feelings of hopelessness, guilt, and sadness.

This activity of the anterior cingulate cortex, however, may tell us something very important. Perhaps we're not reflexively "bad," but rather just "weak" in a way that we don't want to be overwhelmed. We live in a crowded world of seven billion people. If our conscious brain tried to empathize with every person we met, including those experiencing homelessness—to really appreciate their suffering—it would paralyze us. Our ability to empathize needs physiologic brakes.

Los Angeles, San Francisco, and other cities around the nation, including Raleigh, are starting to drown in homelessness. It stands to reason that as the amount of suffering grows, the temptation to use these inherent defense mechanisms will become greater. Walking down the streets of San Francisco or Los Angeles and pausing to consider the humanity of each individual would be overwhelming.

So we don't. Instead, our brains help us out, and as Dr. Harris went on to explain, "dehumanization becomes a sort of emotion regulation strategy."[3] While in the short term, this can allow us to get through our days more easily, in the long term this strategy can prove to be costly, both in terms of human suffering and also the economic efficiency of our social safety nets.

Fortunately, it turns out that the prefrontal cortex is not that hard to activate.

In his subsequent research with England's Museum of Homelessness, Dr. Harris was able to demonstrate that empathy can be quickly triggered—to hold our instinctual predispositions toward judgment and dehumanization in check—by simply pausing to think about the person *as a person*.

As authors Katy Johnston and Hannah Westwater explained in their 2019 article on Dr. Harris's research: "In his experiments, he made participants humanize people by, for example, asking them to consider questions like: 'Does this person prefer broccoli or carrots?' He also scanned people's brain activity before and after speaking to someone sleeping rough. After this kind of interaction, Harris found that participants were far less likely to spontaneously disengage. The medial prefrontal cortexes lit up as those who suffered from homelessness quickly transformed into being seen as humans by the participants. This was simply done by referencing common or shared experiences that make the person relatable—family, kids, likes, hobbies."[4]

This provides a more optimistic picture and points to a practical solution: stop, pause, and humanize. Take a few brief seconds to correct flawed biases and stereotypes, to light up and engage your medial prefrontal cortex.

The antidote to dehumanization is intuitive: *Listen!* Blu nailed it.

Blu died way too early in 2021. Her passing devastated a community that would gather for her memorial services in a park a few weeks later. There, people remembered her words, her smile, her inspiration, and her simple message that she had tattooed in big block letters on her forearm—the same message she would end most of her blog posts with: "Love Wins." Blu was a bright light in the lives of so many who really needed one to help them navigate through the darkness. Her example was her message: Our cognitive minds can override instinct and predispositions toward dehumanization. It just takes practice and, as Blu reminded us of and Dr. Harris proved, listening.

Blu's unique ability to bring dignity and comfort through the simple act of listening reminded me of the examples I was exposed to early in my career.

One of my favorite parts of Tracy Kidder's *Rough Sleepers* was a fellow doctor's description of Jim O'Connell's approach to patients: "I think Jim has an attitude of pre-admiration for the people he does not know yet. His assumption is 'Oh, I'm eventually going to like this person. I will probably find some reason over time to like them. I just happen not to know it yet' … Pre-admiration was something like the opposite of prejudice." I saw Jim do this a hundred times—listening intently to patients. Not talking—just listening, looking for that reason and, usually, finding it quickly.

This quote captures the why behind so much of Jim's success with his most challenging patients—reflexive *humanization*—while most of us go the other way. His filter is set on an assumption of good, in all. And why not? This is what turned his job into an honor instead of a burden. Or perhaps still a burden, but one he carried with joy and determination.

If he or Blu had participated in Dr. Harris's studies back when they were young, I wonder what would have lit up in their functional MRIs. They were wired differently. I'm still not sure how or why—genetically inherent awesomeness, or did they deliberately work to develop these skills over time? Or perhaps elements of both?

As a society, we're bad at listening to one another. As a medical community, we're even worse. There is an old adage in medicine that if we listen to our patients, they will tell us what is wrong with them. Despite all our training around this in our medical education, the evidence—and, if we are honest, probably all of our personal experiences—demonstrate we are not that good at it.

In fact, during the patient history that starts every one of our clinical interactions, studies have demonstrated we can only wait approximately 11 seconds before we feel obligated to interrupt and start talking, likely fulfilling a subconscious need to control and direct that interaction.[5] It does make some sense. With a 15-minute visit production model, our goal is to go in, diagnose, and come up with a treatment plan as quickly as possible—to then move on to the next patient. We need to maintain control and direction to stay on track. This leaves little time to listen and, therefore, to understand.

Listening, humanization, and validation may have little role, if any, in historic fee-for-service medical models. However, as medicine evolves, there's an urgency to understand how they can be foundational to successful value-based care strategies. Callousness, bias, reflexive dehumanization, and associated poor outcomes are costly. They make us much worse at our jobs.

The interactions occurring in our medical system truly are a microcosm of our society and how we, as people, interact with one another: instinct, bias, social hierarchy, love, neglect—all of it. We do not practice medicine in a bubble. The social cognitive related pathologies we find in medicine are the same ones you will find causing dysfunctions throughout society. Imagine the human potential if we all, inside and outside of medicine, worked to follow Jim's example and rewired our predispositions toward reflexive "pre-admiration" instead of judgment and dehumanization—and then, as Blu implored us, we all just *actually* listened to one another.

26
FEEDING THE FIRE WHILE FIGHTING THE FLAME

As population health efforts evolve, one thing becomes clear: Medicine does not, and simply cannot, isolate itself from the communities it serves. Strategies around listening better must be extended from the level of the individual patient-provider interactions to that of how health systems interact with the communities we serve and impact. When we do so, however, we might struggle to accept what we hear, especially when it involves historically marginalized populations.

The American healthcare system has not only historically mismanaged homelessness, but we have also helped to create it.

Michelle was quiet and reserved. She preferred to just keep to herself—typically finding a lower bunk in the corner of the Long Island Shelter in Boston. She would spend most of her time reading.

She had worked in a car repair shop in Pennsylvania for years, living paycheck to paycheck. She was in her early 40s when she woke up one morning sweating and struggling to breathe. She went to the hospital where she was admitted for pneumonia. Her infection was complicated by a parapneumonic effusion, a collection of fluid at the base of her lungs that required a chest tube to drain. A day after her chest tube was placed, the Murphy's Law theme of her hospitalization continued as she developed a blood clot that went to her lungs, further compromising her breathing. It would be a few weeks before she got out of the hospital, in relatively good shape and on a blood thinner her doctors told her to stay on for six months.

Michelle had no insurance. She never thought she would need it, as she was always healthy at baseline. She gambled, confident in her health, as millions of Americans did each year. However she got unlucky and lost.

Upon her release, back at home but still out of work as she fought to regain her strength and breath, the medical bills started to roll in.

"They were almost comical," she would later explain to me. "Nothing I could even come close to paying." Eventually, this resulted in paralyzing debt and associated foreclosure. She suddenly found herself homeless.

"I never thought it was even a possibility until I looked up and realized it was an actual reality," she reflected.

For years, she had avoided drinking like the plague, given that both her mother and father died from complications of alcohol. She also had two brothers who suffered from addiction. With the stress of her new medical issues, homelessness, and associated severe depression, however, she soon found herself drinking heavily. When I got to know her, she still looked back with surprise at just how quickly the addiction hit her.

Without housing and while struggling with her depression and new addiction, her overall health deteriorated. Her chronic medical conditions began to pile up. She started to spend more time in the very hospital where her original wrong turn in life had started. She eventually moved out to Boston where her homelessness, and high healthcare utilization, continued.

Unfortunately, Michelle's story is not uncommon. A $4 trillion-dollar-plus machine will negatively impact the lives of individuals in its path—a lot of individuals. It's inevitable in a nation where many live like Michelle did, paycheck to paycheck, but where the cost of healthcare continues to outpace inflation and wage growth. Between

2010 and 2020, private insurance premiums grew 47 percent. Deductibles grew over 68 percent. Both were significantly higher than both inflation (23 percent) and wage growth (31 percent).[1]

It doesn't take much to knock many Americans over the edge financially, and Michelle's hospital bills were more than enough in her case. Her biggest trauma/anger with the process was the debt collection attempts—aggressive, intimidating, and belittling.

"I was never a leech. Always worked hard and paid my bills. I didn't want to get sick," she reflected one day as she shared her experience with me in clinic.

While hospitals across the nation are increasingly vowing publicly to address health inequities and social barriers of health in the patients they serve, they are simultaneously quietly helping to create them in the poorest members of their community. Some of the wealthiest US hospitals are in communities with the highest debt. Medical debt itself can be a huge social determinant of health that circles back to further exacerbate disparities and inequities, perpetuating the cycle of poverty that contributes to poor health in the first place. Illness often helps to create poverty, and poverty cycles back to worsen illness in what often becomes a deadly positive feedback cycle.

In fact, more than 100 million Americans are faced with medical debt. More than 60 percent of bankruptcies in our country are linked to medical causes—hospital bills, insurance premiums, loss of productivity, and income from illness.[2]

This forces difficult financial decisions—including ones around housing—and further limits access to healthcare by presenting a barrier of fear over returning, even if desperately needed, to the systems a person is indebted to. The current practice of hospitals selling uncollected debt to collection agencies—often bulked, packaged, and sold pennies on the dollar—makes things much worse. Though the debt collection is technically no longer done by the hospitals, the aggressive approaches these companies utilize to collect are still psychologically linked by the patient to the healthcare systems themselves.

For many sick Americans, this entire process can land them,

expensively and dangerously, into homelessness. Foreclosure rates related to medical debt involve racial disparities that cycle back to impact disparities in home ownership and homelessness.[3]

Nobody likes the elephant in the room, but that doesn't mean it's not there. In reality, thousands of sick Americans are likely homeless (and, therefore, sicker) due to medical debt. Fortunately, hospitals nationwide are beginning to partner with nonprofit and community-based organizations to explore how to minimize the impact of medical debt on the most vulnerable members of their communities. There is no one-size-fits-all solution; strategies must be customized to the specific situation and needs of both the hospital and communities they serve.

27

DISPARITIES

If we are to better address homelessness, we will need to understand it in the larger context of health inequities.

Wake County is identical to almost every community in our nation, with data highlighting the health disparities across different neighborhoods. The most economically disadvantaged communities in Wake County are in our southeast neighborhoods. Our census track data, which breaks down information into the more granular neighborhood levels compared to zip code, demonstrates the severity of this poverty and its contrast to other parts of Wake County. In census track 520.1, where WakeMed is headquartered, more than 90 percent of households earn less than twice the federal poverty line threshold. A whopping 36 percent of residents were uninsured before North Carolina's Medicaid expansion in late 2023 —four times the national average.[1] The vast majority of residents are Black.

Knowing that the primary drivers of health outcomes are the social determinants, situations, and environments patients encounter in their daily lives during the 99.9 percent of the time they're not in our hospitals or clinics, the correlating healthcare disparity data is not surprising. Black residents in Wake County, compared to White residents, have an approximately two times higher rate of prostate cancer mortality, three times the rate of death related to both diabetes and kidney disease, and a 34 percent increase in breast-cancer-related mortality. When COVID hit locally, Black residents experienced both a higher infection and mortality rate.[2] The cumulative impact of all these data points contributes to likely the most sobering statistic of all: A person who lives in southeast Raleigh has an average life expectancy that is approximately 12 years less than a person who lives in Raleigh's northwest suburbs.[3]

Looking at most large cities across the nation, you'll see similar patterns of socioeconomic data paralleling health disparity data. You'll also recognize it in America's homeless data where Black individuals are overrepresented by nearly a factor of three compared with the general population.[4] In Wake County, unfortunately, we're just slightly worse than national trends, with almost 70 percent of our homeless community being Black compared to only 20 percent of our general population.[5]

In studying this data, it again becomes clear that any discussions around the root causes of US homelessness and its associated health outcomes can and should be part of larger conversations around health—and social—equity. In many ways, homelessness, especially when chronic, is the ultimate health inequity—the end result or downstream symptom of poorly controlled medical, social, and behavioral health issues that advance and worsen over time, unassisted by systems that, in theory, could and should be helping but instead are focused more on other populations.

Health inequities occur when patients from populations who are socially or economically disadvantaged aren't afforded equal opportunities and possibilities for good health. They have become inevitable consequences of our historic fee-for-service healthcare system that focused on fixing the broken—especially in those who can afford it—instead of promoting health. It's hard to argue that our nation's healthcare system has offered equal opportunities to the socially or economically disadvantaged. When poverty has driven the broken and the deteriorating within communities, health systems have not proactively jumped in to minimize the harm. Public health officials often tried, but they were largely ignored by healthcare systems focused on, and distracted by, maximizing profits elsewhere.

Enter value-based care—determined to "bend the cost curve" of healthcare. In 2015, the percentage of value-based payments—reimbursement determined by quality and cost metrics instead of simply volume—was 23 percent. In 2021, it was over 40 percent.[6] The current goal is to move 100 percent of Medicare and Medicaid to value-based payment models by 2030,[7] with commercial payers expected to continue to follow.

As we pivot toward getting reimbursed for how we maximize health instead of how we fix the broken, medical providers are working to better understand the true underlying factors that drive poor patient outcomes, including the deep-seated health inequities in our communities.

A woman was filling out a form at a COVID-19 vaccine event I was helping to staff. Usually people try to speed through the required demographic questions and just sign the consent. However, she paused, reflecting, "I always get caught up on this question. I'm considered Black, but only my dad's dad is Black. My other three grandparents are White. But I guess I am considered Black."

In 2017, a patient brought his DNA profile from a commercial vendor to his annual physical. He was a White man raised on a farm in Louisiana, thick accent and all. He was surprised to discover he had 10 percent "Sub-Saharan Africa DNA." A few months later, in a similar occurrence, a patient who considered herself "100 percent Black" found that she had more than 12 percent European DNA.

They were both shocked. They should not have been.

The 2003 Human Genome Project demonstrated humans are 99.9 percent identical at the DNA level. Genetic exchanges that occurred through migration, trade, conquests, and other historical events have ensured that the remaining 0.1 percent is a universal mix displayed in these DNA assessments found in the market.[8]

At the individual level, to attempt to assign races across this spectrum of inherent genetic variability, especially down to just a few possible selections, is, by definition, arbitrary. Race is ambiguous—attempts to force it into the unambiguous go against science.

Dr. Rasheeda Monroe tells about a case of a Black child with breathing issues. Diagnostically, the team had become stuck when trying to identify a cause for his symptoms. As the team presented the case, facts scribbled on the whiteboard and chest X-ray on display, a radiologist strolled into the room, quickly looked at the X-ray, and said, "Cystic fibrosis." Nobody had thought about it—less than 5 percent of cystic fibrosis is in Black patients—yet after he said it, looking at the chest X-ray, it was obvious. Sometimes life (and genetics and medicine) is not black and white. Or not nearly to the extent we think.

Race and ethnicity can undoubtedly be associated with an increase in the prevalence of certain diseases or health conditions, such as sickle cell anemia or cystic fibrosis itself. But this concept of race as a biological determinant of disease is complex, often oversimplified, and dangerously misunderstood in medicine.

The link between race and health disparities is likely much more influenced by social and environmental stressors that flood bodies with pathological levels of cortisol than by genetics (although the recent field of epigenetics demonstrates how stress can impact genetics themselves—which is likely a whole other book).

It is often the marginalization itself, and its stress-related physiologic harm, that drives the poor outcomes of the "historically marginalized."

Yet we too often fall into the trap of focusing solely on race, mistakenly attributing poor patient outcomes to simplistic categorical risk factors that do not truly exist. It's easier to do so, but it's also wrong. By doing so, we miss the opportunities to better address the *actual* root causes that lie in communities we serve outside of the walls of our clinics and hospitals. These causes include a lack of social capital, economic mobility, housing, employment, and educational opportunities —all of which are often rooted in the pervasive dehumanization and associated racism that gives rise to social inequities, disparities, trauma, and ACEs themselves.

A recent analysis by Deloitte looked at the high annual cost of health inequities: an estimated $326 billion currently, projected to be at $1 billion by 2040.[9] In medicine, there is typically a financial cost that directly correlates to the human cost. The data that drives and directs value-based care will continue to shine a bright light on health inequities in a way that cannot continue to be ignored.

In its *ideal* form, value-based care will only focus on and incentivize health to try to minimize the cost of poor health to the extent possible. It will be too expensive not to do so. We are far from any pure or ideal model, but as value-based care evolves, a productive sense of urgency will lead us to better understand and address the root causes of poor health outcomes in order to minimize their financial impact. Inevitably, this will result in health systems becoming more involved with issues of social justice, if they are increasingly held accountable for the costly health outcomes of social *in*justice. This will move systems beyond the simple provision of transportation, food boxes, or even housing units in high-risk individuals—to address identified social determinants of health (symptoms)—to more intentional efforts and strategies around social injustices (root causes). Not necessarily owning efforts, but collaborating with local partners and social sectors to improve the communities they serve. This won't be partisan or political; it won't even necessarily be advocacy. It will be strategy.

Chronic homelessness is often a symptom, not a root cause—a deadly downstream manifestation of a lifetime (or generations) of environmental stress, disproportionately affecting historically marginalized populations. If we hope to efficiently address the worsening crisis of homelessness in America, it will truly take a village.

PART V
SHARED ROOTS

Dehumanization at the level of our individual interactions with those experiencing homelessness is generalized into our societal approaches to chronic homelessness. Our desire to avoid empathy, often facilitated through blame, serves a similar function at both the societal and individual levels: It demands less effort, causes less discomfort, and spares us from worry. Our lives become easier, and we can move on despite the dysfunction and its associated high costs.

The deep-seated roots of dehumanization around homelessness spread across social sectors outside of just medicine and underlie the hypocritical gaps between our professed political and religious ideals and our actual actions.

If we better understand what drives these gaps, we can better address them—as we strive to live up to the shared values and beliefs that, if we are smart, should unite us as a nation.

28

MENTAL HEALTH

Evan was a patient I cared for at my Long Island clinic in Boston. He was a participant in the facility's reentry program, designed to help recently incarcerated homeless patients reassimilate into society. He'd just gotten out of prison after 40 years. I followed him in clinic to help stabilize his chronic diabetes and hypertension.

In his late 50s, he looked like he'd been cast right out of Hollywood—bald head, crooked nose, gruffly voice. However, he was both articulate and friendly. He would often come up to the clinic just to socialize.

Evan grew up in a large Boston family—one of many boys and one sister. He was in the middle of the pack, the third oldest. His mother left them early. He explained he was "not sure why, but imagine I couldn't blame her." His father had a quick and violent temper. "He would beat the crap out of all of us equally." His oldest brother was his role model and often attempted to protect his younger siblings, "trying to take the brunt of the beatings."

One night, Evan came home "on cloud nine" after making his middle-school varsity basketball team, looking to celebrate and brag to his brothers. His father, especially intoxicated that night, was angry that Evan came home late. Evan's beating that night was particularly brutal. As he fell to the ground, his father didn't let up—continuing to kick him in the face and chest. His oldest brother ran to protect him, sparing Evan from the continued rage by redirecting the violence to himself. His father choked his brother until he passed out. Evan thought his brother was dead as his dad staggered out the door.

Evan battled through that childhood and was determined to attend community college when it happened. Fast and sudden, and over before he knew it. An argument with a neighborhood friend "over nothing important" while they were both drinking, although Evan recalled he was only one to two beers in at the time. Evan snapped, grabbing a knife, and blindly, in a rage, stabbed the teen three times, once through the heart. His friend ended up dying, and Evan ended up behind bars for 40 years with nightly flashbacks of the events of that evening that would haunt him for the rest of his life.

Evan had known his friend's family well. His parents had helped support Evan through his tough childhood, and his little sister was a good friend of Evan's. Evan blamed his PTSD after the event as much on "the way his parents looked at me in court" as the stabbing itself. Interestingly, he did not even really remember his own father's reaction.

He was tormented by the loss of potential—both in his friend's life and in his own.

He had fought hard his whole life. He'd stayed clean, determined.

"Four seconds, and just like that, it was gone"

He reflected, "I am still in shock that I had it in me. I'm not a violent guy. I just snapped. That is what has been killing me for 40 years."

Evan spent his decades of incarceration isolated without any visits from family or friends. His oldest brother died a few years before he got out of prison. While Evan thought his brother knew that he loved and appreciated him, he was not sure if he'd ever actually told him this directly.

One evening, Evan came up to the clinic to ask for advice on how to mail a letter. He'd never mailed one before. With only slight embarrassment, he pulled out a folded envelope. He had placed the address correctly in the center (without the zip code, however) but had misplaced the stamp in the bottom right corner.

"I had no idea," he shrugged as I corrected it. "Never done it before."

Four seconds resulting in 40 years of missed opportunities and life. Could there be anything more tormenting? But there he was, in my clinic—smiling the best he could, learning the best he could, as he worked to salvage the rest of his life the best he could. Speaker and author Ed Mylett once stated that "the most inspiring person is the one overcoming the fear of doing something, not the person who is excellent at it."

Evan was definitely "not good at life," but he was desperately trying to get better.

Earlier that evening, I'd called my wife on my way to the shelter, complaining about how busy work had been over the past few weeks. After hearing Evan's story, it would be a while before I complained about anything again.

So much of life is about how we use our cognition to control our emotions, instincts, and predispositions. How we think instead of just reacting to a world that is constantly reacting to us. How we use our prefrontal cortex to filter and control the reactive parts of our brain.

So many of life's hardships can result from *not* being able to do so—when a person's cognitive abilities and efforts are overwhelmed by their circumstances. This is especially true when one's world is particularly harsh, violent, unfair, and toxic. It can be extremely challenging, but think of all the crimes, divorces, acts of violence, addiction relapses, and suffering that could be avoided if people were more empowered to control emotions and anger. Destroyed relationships, careers, and potential. Explosions and fights and so much that is detrimental to our lives—all circling back to be sources of continued and mounting levels of stress and misery and more trauma. This is something that many of my patients have reflected on in my discussions with them about trauma and its impact. "If only I had not done ..." "If only if I had not reacted."

Instinctual acts of rage and emotion are often the devastating downstream, life-impacting results of historic trauma and ACEs. So much pain and suffering can be traced back to the cognitive inability to control overpowering emotion and impulse—the very skill that historic trauma anatomically compromises. Underdeveloped prefrontal cortexes predispose to poor impulse control while overdeveloped amygdalae and ventral medial hypothalamuses misinterpret threats and trigger anxiety and reactivity.

Empowering patients to better control emotions, rage, and instinct is essential in helping to minimize the damaging effects of trauma. It can also help break its devastating trans-generational cycles.

Those who suffer from the trauma inflicted on them by others are often predisposed to inflict it on others. Victims become perpetrators. A child who grows up in an environment of addiction and violence is more likely to suffer from addictions and force violence on others as they age.[1,2] The most dangerous characteristic of the pathology of trauma is this ability to evolve its victims into its future hosts. It's a messy, expensive and viral-like cycle that spreads through generations.

The best way to break the disease cycle, like any virus, is to treat the current victim to halt the future spread.

But how do we do this? How do we empower patients to cognitively control emotions? This is the million-dollar (or multi-billion- ... trillion-dollar?) question in medicine. It is *the* foundational goal of mental health therapy, for patients both with and without trauma.

People will pay hundreds of dollars an hour to lie on couches and learn the hidden secrets on how to do this. Increasingly, it seems you cannot learn those secrets *without* paying those hundreds of dollars per hour.

For years now, I've struggled to get my patients in to see mental health providers—even those patients with commercial insurance but who still suffer from poverty. Due to high copays associated with specialists, and availability, my patients (and I) have almost stopped trying, which forces them (and I) into settling for me not only serving as their primary care provider but also frequently as their psychiatrist and therapist.

I am not alone in this. Other primary care physicians around the nation are having to do the same.

It's estimated that in a general population for good mental healthcare, you need about 15 psychiatrists per 100,000 people—and this was pre-COVID and before the growing social media explosion that is wreaking havoc on people's mental health. A 2018 analysis demonstrated we were at 9 psychiatrists per 100,000. An astonishing 60 percent of US counties had no practicing psychiatrists at all.[3]

A few years ago, researchers in California called 229 psychiatrists listed in the *Los Angeles County Super Pages*. They described themselves as "a person with serious mental health symptoms who needed a medication evaluation." Only 28 were actually able to make an appointment. Eighty percent had a wait time of over five weeks (a lot of poor mental health outcomes can happen in that time). The medium consult fee: $450.[4]

Many psychiatrists have cited both the reductions in payments and administrative burdens as reasons why they have stopped taking insurance. One thing I learned in my seven years as chief medical officer of our ACO is that insurance companies are slow to adapt to anything. I think even insurance companies would agree. There is an increasing amount of data highlighting the importance of mental health on physical health outcomes and related cost. However, as the central importance of mental health in an evolving value-based model becomes more apparent, the reimbursements for that care don't support its value—not even close.

A Congressional Budget Office study done in 2019 found that US commercial insurance plans had average in-network rates for common mental health services that were 13 percent to 14 percent *less* than traditional Medicare fee-for-service rates in traditional Medicare.[5] This number highlights how misaligned priorities are, especially when you consider that commercial rates for other outpatient and physician services are often well over 50 percent *higher* than Medicare.[6] As a result, many mental health providers have stopped taking insurance altogether—because they can—and do what cosmetic surgeons and other elective procedure-type providers have done for years: cash pay, for patients who can afford it. In a 2014 Weill Cornell Medical College study published in *JAMA Psychiatry*, about 45 percent of psychiatrists didn't accept private health insurance or Medicaid.[7] The rest often accept a limited number of plans. Therapists are following suit. No insurance red tape—just cash, and a lot of it.[8]

We have never done mental health well in this nation. In fact, according to a 2017 Kaiser study, the US has "the highest mortality rate for these disorders among similarly wealthy countries."[9] As behavioral health access continues to deteriorate, associated poor mental health outcomes are disproportionately affecting poorer populations. Any time demand for a need exceeds supply, you will inevitably start to see a disparity in utilization between those who can afford it and those who cannot. As many behavioral health providers leverage this favorable supply/demand ratio into cash-only reimbursements, poor and historically marginalized populations have increasingly been priced out of access. Those who continue to take insurance are often incentivized to cherry-pick away from patients with the most severe pathologies, as the relatively small reimbursements simply aren't worth the extra time needed to control their complicated pathologies.

Those suffering from homelessness are on the bottom, losing ends of those disparities, with their often-severe mental health pathologies expensively and dangerously ignored. This not only compromises our ability to manage mental illness in individuals already experiencing chronic homelessness, but also in those who are newly homeless, increasing the likelihood that they get expensively trapped in its chronic form. Those who need mental healthcare the most are being left without resources; it's a familiar story in the history of American medicine that we're working to evolve away from, yet we find ourselves handcuffed by a behavioral health world that is simultaneously going in the opposite direction. The supply isn't even close to matching the demand.

As we're increasingly focused on controlling costs in sick populations, we're learning just how costly a lack of access to behavioral health can be.

In 2020, the consulting firm, Milliman, released a study that assessed the impact of behavioral health on overall medical cost by analyzing the commercial insurance claims of more than 21 million people. The results were stunning … kind of.

Researchers once again identified the familiar pattern of a small percentage of patients being responsible for the majority of the cost; here, 10 percent of the population was responsible for 70 percent of the total healthcare cost. The average annual medical costs for this "top 10 percent"? $41,631—more than 20 times higher than the $1,965 annual cost of the bottom 90 percent.

Of the 2.1 million people who made up this highest-cost 10 percent of patients, 57 percent suffered from behavioral health issues. This small subset of 1.2 million patients, or 5.7 percent of the total 21 million patient cohort, was responsible for 44 percent of the total cost. Yet half of these highest-cost patients with behavioral health issues spent less than $95 per year on mental health treatment. Overall, those patients with mental health conditions spent 2.8 to 6.2 times more for their medical care.[10]

Commercial payers and their employer customers have blindly hemorrhaged money dealing with medical symptoms, while expensively ignoring the mental health issues that are often root causes.

I found the Milliman study so intriguing that I had our ACO coordinate a webinar on the topic with one of the study's authors, Steve Melek, a few months through the *American Journal of Managed Care*. During the webinar, Steve reflected, "The takeaway is that people with behavioral conditions use a lot of healthcare. A significant majority of the total healthcare costs come from people that have a behavioral disorder and very often it's comorbid with chronic medical conditions." He emphasized "the importance of … getting behavioral health available to people who commonly have physical health conditions."[11]

It's pretty simple: If you want to better control medical costs, invest in mental health.

We did just that in our hotspotter model at WakeMed. As an internal medicine physician, I knew I was in over my head with trying to manage our highest-risk patients whose medical issues were driven by complex mental illness. It became clear that evolving population health models needed more behavioral health guidance and leadership if we were to improve outcomes. In 2017, we secured two grants that allowed us the opportunity to achieve this.

Dr. Nerissa Price is the daughter of a teacher and a pastor. She grew up in the same zip code as WakeMed, attending North Carolina State University as an undergraduate prior to going to the University of North Carolina for medical school. She has dedicated her career to community psychiatry, with a particular interest in the most complicated and historically neglected populations. She has worked in prisons, community clinics, and the streets, proactively seeking out patients who need the most help—those whose mental illness is often so severe, involving paranoia and suspicions, that they won't seek help themselves.

She joined our team in 2018 to lead both a new, grant-funded, dedicated behavioral health case management team as well as a homeless street outreach team funded through a separate federal grant. The latter was designed to proactively engage unsheltered individuals with severe mental and persistent mental illness. They didn't necessarily have heavy utilization of healthcare resources. In fact, many refused to seek out medical attention even when they desperately needed it. Their disabling and sometimes paralyzing mental illnesses kept them isolated and hidden, often deep in the woods. Dr. Price and her team, led by Dr. Arlene Smith, would engage and build trust with unsheltered homeless residents, working to get them access to mental illness treatment and, ideally, housing. We believed this outreach team would provide a balance to our otherwise heavy focus on high utilizers identified through analytics.

Over the years, we continued to gain experience with these models as we leveraged Dr. Price's expertise and knowledge to evolve how we better addressed severe mental illness, both inside, but just as importantly, outside, our medical silos. This included developing different trauma-informed teams and processes for our patients that included both group and individual therapy approaches. It also meant building collaborative care models for our highest-risk patients.

For me clinically, it provided access to psychiatry for patients with the most severe cases of mental illnesses that no community behavioral health provider would be willing to see unless they were more stable. Over the years, we had extreme difficulties getting any outpatient *mental health* providers to see our patients with actual severe mental health. We tried but constantly failed.

The reasons we received back from our local mental health providers?

They were late. They were aggressive toward staff. They never answered their phones. They were intoxicated. They were disorganized. They never filled out forms.

The chaotic manifestations of the very illnesses we were trying to get them help for, which were often dangerously raging out of control, were the actual barriers that prevented their own care. Nobody was running toward these patients to help, fearing if they did, they would get stuck managing them. So instead, there was shoulder shrugging, dismissing, and barring instead of helping them through what, ultimately, were clinical manifestations of their diseases.

Dr. Price would see, stabilize, and help advocate to place these sicker patients into long-term mental health homes.

We were fortunate that we had the resources to include psychiatry support in our models. However, on a larger scale, the reality remains clear: There is no cavalry of benevolent mental health providers coming to save the day by altruistically making financial sacrifices to serve the historically marginalized populations as they suffer disproportionately from mental health issues. If those providers can continue hanging out on their therapy couches with patients who can dish out $200-plus an hour in cash—avoiding the under-reimbursed hassle of dealing with insurance companies while working on their easier issues like youth-soccer-team-placement injustices instead of severe, crippling trauma and addiction—why wouldn't they? The hero model is never a sustainable public health strategy.

Unless we (quickly) evolve reimbursement models to sufficiently compensate mental health providers for the challenging, yet vital, work of helping to address mental health in our highest risk and most challenging patients, mental health will continue to drive and worsen our current national crisis around chronic homelessness. As we push for payment reform, we need to simultaneously answer the following question: If the behavioral health market has, to a large extent, priced out poor and historically marginalized populations—the very people who need it the most—how do we do the best we can with our current realities?

(See Appendix 2: Patient Insight, Not Labels and Appendix 3: Creating More Efficient and Accessible Mental Health Tools for Historically Marginalized Populations.)

29

JUSTICE SYSTEM

I once had a patient go to the emergency room with diabetic ketoacidosis. In fact, I've likely had hundreds. But let's call this particular patient Joe ... or Sharon.

Joe/Sharon showed up with very high blood sugars that resulted in acidosis, a dangerous consequence of the body's inability to effectively draw sugar out of the blood and into cells for metabolism. It's potentially deadly if not treated appropriately by effectively addressing the underlying pathology of insulin deficiency. So typically, we identify and treat it by giving the body the insulin it's lacking. We've become good at managing this condition in medicine. Just over a hundred years ago, we didn't know what diabetic ketoacidosis really was. Today, we identify and effectively manage it on a daily basis in our community emergency rooms, saving patients' lives by efficiently addressing a life-threatening pathology. This is awesome and exactly what we should be doing in medicine.

Now imagine if, when Joe/Sharon presented to the ER with diabetic ketoacidosis, we didn't treat them. We didn't give them insulin. That would obviously be negligent. But now imagine if when they presented sick, we actually hooked them up to an IV Kool-Aid drip instead of an IV insulin drip. How ineffective, costly, and dangerous would it be to actually *exacerbate* the underlying presenting pathology instead of treating it? Suffering would increase, followed by potential death and an associated high cost. We would clearly be violating our obligation to effectively treat patients to the best of our abilities.

Yet this is exactly what we routinely do, in and out of our hospitals, with people who have mental health issues and a history of trauma.

There is perhaps no greater, or more dangerous and expensive, display of our inefficiencies—addressing both homelessness and mental health—than what is found behind the bars of our prisons and jails.

When it comes to the interface of medicine and the justice system, with patients suffering from mental illness, our story in this country is one of mutual failure and IV Kool-Aid drips. Medicine often fails to effectively manage pathologies of mental health, trauma, and addiction, allowing their symptomatic manifestations to land people in jails and prisons. Upon release, these conditions are typically not well treated. Patients are rarely well connected with mental health care that would minimize the chance of dangerous, and expensive, recidivism. What ensues are revolving doors of inefficiency that further exacerbate pathologies and prevent an individual's social progress and success.

Frequent incarcerations and run-ins with law enforcement are common barriers to social and financial progress and improved health in unhoused individuals, or more broadly, in people from lower socioeconomic status. Incarcerations are often the "two-steps-back" in life that negate any one-step-forward in social advancement an individual may have fought to accomplish.

Studies have demonstrated approximately 15 percent of all incarcerated people were homeless in the year prior to their incarceration,[1] a much higher rate than in the general population, which hovers around 0.2 percent.[2] On the other hand, people with a history of any sort of incarceration are 13 times more likely to be homeless compared to the general public.[3,4] The similar rates of overrepresentation of people of color in both the justice system and homelessness populations is no coincidence.

Much of this criminal activity in the homeless population involves public "nuisance" offenses related to the daily realities of homelessness. The daily activities of living that most of us do in the privacy of our homes—urinating, sleeping, drinking, changing clothes—are considered criminal acts when done outdoors by people without homes. Indeed, rates of interactions with the criminal systems of unsheltered homeless residents living outside are higher than those living in the shelters.[5]

In April of 2020, when COVID hit and homeless shelters reduced capacity, our outreach team went out to homeless campsites to help provide food, hygiene supplies, and simple education about the pandemic. Yet when we went to one of the largest sites our team frequently visited, we found it abandoned. We discovered that police had shut it down a few days earlier, placing signs that it was illegal to lodge or sleep outside in that location. While tucked away deep in a wooded area, the site was large enough to draw significant traffic, which apparently resulted in complaints from local residents. When our outreach team showed up that day, all that was left were piles of trash. Nobody remained. The same people being turned away from homeless shelters due to space limitations related to social distancing were now being told it was illegal to stay outside—even in areas hidden deep and isolated.

We naturally asked ourselves, "Where are they supposed to go?" Our patients would ask us this same question countless times in the following months. Campsites and "tent cities" were set up, only to be shut down by law enforcement. While we were all sheltering in place, homelessness was being exacerbated, and at the same time, criminalized in our communities. While our specific community did an excellent job of quickly and effectively providing hotel options for the oldest and sickest people suffering from homelessness, many more were left without options. The demand was too great.

In addition to these crimes of existence, society's struggles to effectively manage mental health conditions, as discussed in the previous chapter, also drive the disproportionately higher incarceration rates in homeless individuals. As medicine fails to effectively help chronically homeless individuals suffering from mental illness, the symptomatic manifestations of these pathologies in the community frequently result in interactions with the criminal justice system. Hallucinations, delusions, mania, and agitation frequently get expressed in illegal activities.

Our nation has a historically punitive justice system with one of the highest incarceration rates in the world.[79] It's based on the concept of an individual's accountability for their actions; by design, it's set up to punish the act, not necessarily the person. It typically doesn't attempt to understand, nor take into account, the historical drivers of the actions it punishes, including those related to trauma or mental health, except in its extreme forms. It doesn't incorporate arguments of neuroanatomic pathologies. For example, the violent actions of a person with antisocial personality disorder may be related to (inflexible?) impairments in a prefrontal-temporal-limbic system,[6] but this typically isn't used in legal arguments.

In prison populations, research has identified that 97 percent of the population have one adverse childhood event, with a staggering 78.1 percent having four or more.[7] So many crimes of reaction or reflexive rage are likely driven by a lack of impulse control, yet these traumatic childhood experiences that can neurobiologically predispose someone toward criminal acts aren't routinely part of legal arguments.

This approach helps us maintain some objectivity directed at the criminal action itself, while avoiding the slippery slope of relative subjectivity that would be introduced if we tried to psychoanalyze the typically complicated reasons behind those actions. Every action we engage in, really, is the result of the cumulative impact of all our lifetime experiences and acts that led us to that point—which is an impossibly complex process. A foundational aspect of our justice system is that actions themselves have consequences for which people must be held accountable; this makes sense on multiple levels.

Our justice system is designed to punish, but not rehabilitate—and therefore to often exacerbate, but not treat.

In the isolation and dead time of jails and prisons, the very pathologies responsible for the criminal act in the first place continue to progress. Social isolation drives stress and maladaptive social strategies. It exacerbates pathologies of the limbic system of the brain. It leads to more agitation and aggression. It results in worsening depression and anxiety and provides an environment that further dehumanizes those incarcerated. In fact, dehumanization is not just a consequence of incarceration's punishment; it *is* the punishment. Social isolation, small cells, standard uniforms, number assignments. My patients who have been incarcerated often share the same experience as the former captives I have served in Hostage US. It's often the dehumanization associated with incarcerations that they perceive to be the most traumatizing part of their experience.

This toxic environment of stress and dehumanization serves as the IV Kool-Aid drip for many of the underlying pathologies that led to the incarceration.

Upon their release from jail and prison, people are rarely well connected to the help they need to have a chance at good health and successful outcomes. Any connections to mental health or medical resources that may have existed prior to incarceration are typically not reestablished, and access to important psychiatric medications is often limited.

Too often in our shelters and day programs, we see people dropped off after being released from jail or prison. They are off medications with no follow-up appointments, no guidance, and no connections to help them meet basic needs.

One cold night when I was working at the overnight shelter during COVID, I met a young Black man in his 20s who had been transported to the shelter straight from prison earlier that afternoon. At the time, jails and prisons were trying to reduce overcrowding in order to help control the spread of COVID. He asked me if there was any way he could get clothes. He was dropped off in just a T-shirt, shoes with no laces (shoelaces are often taken away during entry into jail as a suicide prevention measure), and no idea where to go the next day. No resources.

"I'm lost," he said. "I have no idea where to start tomorrow." Then he paused to add, "Damn, it's cold outside."

He left the next day at 8 a.m., as we were closing—in the freezing rain, with a hat, socks, and jacket we were able to find for him, but without shoelaces, an umbrella, or a sense of dignity ... or hope. He trudged through large puddles, alone and soaked, with written directions we had given him to access Oak City Cares with the bus. I haven't seen him since.

For those released from incarceration, this lack of connection to medical and behavioral health treatment, combined with the housing and job discrimination associated with criminal records, further perpetuates the nightmare of homelessness. People are hopelessly steered back toward continued criminal acts of necessity and reaction. The result is often inevitable recidivism—costly and dangerous. It's no surprise that two-thirds of the 650,000 people released from prison annually are arrested again within three years.[8,9] This reinforces an expensive cycle of tax-funded dysfunction. It's often unproductively punitive and exacerbating instead of innovatively rehabilitative.

This cycle of inevitable recidivism and dysfunction can be particularly damaging in younger populations. As children who experience trauma transition to becoming young adults, their pathologies can become less sympathy-provoking and potentially more dangerous and criminal. Incarcerations and interactions with the judicial system are often the early flames that can ignite the fuel built up by adverse childhood experiences, quickly consuming and destroying any potential for success in early adulthood.

Many young people may not have the support, financial or social, to successfully get back on their feet after initial incarcerations. Post-incarceration homelessness and social struggles can quickly snowball into a cycle of chronic dysfunction. Common homeless-related, non-violent crimes can build criminal records and shrink employment and housing opportunities, paving a direct path to chronic and sustained homelessness. This slippery slope can form quickly. Studies have demonstrated that while people with one incarceration are more than seven times more likely to suffer from homelessness compared to the general population, this almost doubles to 13 times higher with two or more. Recidivism builds on recidivism, labels accumulating ("felon," "repeat offender," "homeless")—the Kool-Aid IV drip exacerbating. One early mistake or offense can quickly avalanche into a life of costly hardships, suffering, and homelessness.

Any intervention or treatment that circles back to worsen the issue that it's trying to address, by definition, must be judged as counterproductive and counterintuitive. While our punitive justice system, in theory, works to increase accountability in those it encounters, it has historically perpetuated an expensive inefficiency that compromises public safety through exacerbating mental illness.

Trauma on top of trauma. Pathologies exacerbated, not treated. Formulas for costly and inevitably bad outcomes are dangerous for those incarcerated as well as the society they interact with.

It simply becomes an argument of efficiency to develop more rehabilitative-focused strategies that better address trauma, and focus on safe discharges with less chance of recidivism. It makes sense to minimize the link between incarcerations and homelessness by better connecting people exiting jails and prisons to community and healthcare resources—to provide opportunities for success for those with frequent interactions with the justice system due to lack of opportunities, and poorly controlled pathologies. Address the underlying causes; don't exacerbate them.

The first, relatively intuitive step in justice reform for those experiencing homelessness is to resolve "crimes of living" offenses through practical solutions instead of expensive jail time. This would involve linking "offenders" to necessary assistance instead of counterproductive, punitive incarceration that worsens root causes and expensively increases pressure on our overburdened judicial system.

In 1993, San Diego developed the nation's first "homeless court." Special court sessions were convened in the city's homeless shelters that allowed defendants to resolve misdemeanors and minor offenses. Since that time, more than 70 communities from around the nation have adopted this model.[10]

The second, more complicated step is when people do end up in our jails and prisons, let's start to better address the mental health and pathologies that landed them there in the first place. If our prisons and jails in America are truly our nation's largest mental health facilities, let's accept this reality in an effort to stop this cycle of expensive dysfunction. Nobody—especially an offender—wants to see people who are incarcerated return after they are released. While these pathologies can be complex and overwhelming, as can be their treatment, we can at least start to improve how we address them. Perfect is the enemy of good. Just start with better.

This doesn't necessarily require a complete overhaul of our historic justice and punitive system. It can start with an improved insight into neurobiology, trauma, and pathology—incorporating trauma-informed models, not as a demonstration of enlightenment, but as strategies to improve efficiency of prison and jail management by lowering predispositions to recidivism.

How can we work with individuals to help them build the cognitive control and processing of emotions that likely keeps most of us from landing in jail? We need more individualized therapy and health education to empower those incarcerated. What drives them to commit criminal actions? How can they develop skills around impulse control? How can they control the reflexives of rage, anger, fear, or anxiety that they later regret? As our understanding of human behavior continues to evolve, we'll find more ways to efficiently assist patients with these predispositions toward criminal acts. We must build this as a continuum for their eventual reentry into society. Upon release from incarceration, reconnection to medical, behavioral health, and social resources should be an essential component in minimizing recidivism. Fortunately, "reentry" programs designed to do just that have started throughout the country.

This work has been pioneered locally in North Carolina by Dr. Evan Ashkin and his team at the University of North Carolina. He designed the Formerly Incarcerated Transitions (FIT) program to help recently incarcerated men and women to avoid the common pitfalls and barriers to success upon their release. His motivations for addressing issues resulting in recidivism are as economic as they are humane. "The fact that economically we let it be this way is just another example of how much bias and prejudice there is in this system, that we don't connect people to basic care."[11] The foundation of the FIT Program is the team's community health workers who have lived experiences of incarceration. They share their experiences in an effort to help navigate their clients through the confusing and complex safety nets of medical, behavioral, and social services to get the care they need to be successful. The FIT program has demonstrated decreased recidivism and associated cost savings, helping to prove the intuitive: that insulin works much better than Kool-Aid.

As the growing crisis of homelessness threatens to cripple cities, counties, and communities nationwide, and with our jails and prison expensively overcrowded in a nation with the sixth highest incarceration rate in the world, this is a critical lesson to pay attention to.[12]

30

ONE NATION

If we want to improve the efficiency and humanity of how we manage the worsening crisis around homelessness in the US, we will need legislative support to drive innovative solutions across various social sectors. This can only be achieved through thoughtful political debate on how to evolve our policies based on evidence, experience, and a better understanding of chronic homelessness.

The problem: We've become really bad at "thoughtful political debate." The root cause behind this is familiar.

We all have more in common than we do not. Deep down, I think we all realize this. But in a deteriorating political environment, where both sides intentionally manipulate conflict and disagreement for political gain, this is increasingly being forgotten. As political efforts to weaponize ourselves against one other grow, collaboration and agreement are increasingly rare in our government, both at the local and national levels. The historical use of political discourse to guide the best path for society has been hijacked by the self-serving interests of those working to gain power, votes, or simple clicks, so you'll watch a 15-second GEICO commercial prior to their divisive clip. Their primary strategy is both lazy and, if you study history, extremely predictable: dehumanization of "the other."

Ad hominem, directing an argument or reaction against another person rather than on their position on the debated topic, has historically been viewed as unacceptable, or at least unprofessional, in political discourse. And for good reason—it dumbs down our political conversations and therefore our society as a whole. An element of ad hominem has always snuck into politics. Recently, however, it has gotten much worse. At this point, people seem to have stopped even trying to disguise it. Thoughtful discussion has been replaced with blatant and routine character assassination. The focus is not to debate those with opposing views to yours in an effort to find common ground to guide the best path forward; it's to "cancel" them. It deteriorates the contemplative into the reactive. And, when *reactive* is reacting against *reactive*, especially at the level of political discourse in government, things tend to not go too well … or at least much worse than if *contemplative* is contemplating with *contemplative*. Battling amygdalae rarely lead to productive outcomes. Engaged prefrontal cortexes do.

This deteriorating political and societal climate increasingly obscures the common ideals of respect, justice, altruism, or just basic decency—preached from the different pulpits, living room couches, classrooms, and boardrooms in our nation—into something no longer recognizable. Historically, one such commonly shared ideal was the sense of calling, or even obligation, to assist those in our communities who can't fully care for themselves. You can tell a lot about a society by how it actually accomplishes this—both from a humanistic and, perhaps more importantly, from an efficiency perspective. Human suffering is expensive. Avoidable human suffering is wasteful.

While most people resonate with this idea of assisting those who can't fully help themselves, the disagreements shaping the political divide often focus on the extent to which a person actually *is* capable of caring for themselves. The humanistic desire to provide charity and assistance for those who need it is understandably balanced by concern around the potential for expensive enablement and dependency of the "able-bodied" who are simply "milking the system."

Even in today's polarized environment, few would argue against the need for society to help an 85-year-old woman suffering from advancing Alzheimer's who is wandering the streets in confusion. Or a 25-year-old male with Down's Syndrome who recently lost both parents. There's general acceptance that these conditions prevent their brains from navigating them safely through daily life. Both Alzheimer's and Down's Syndrome are well studied and understood; we know their mechanisms. This understanding then triggers our sense of obligation to assist.

The pathophysiology and biology of mental health, addiction, and trauma—which frequently underlie chronic homelessness—are far less understood, although their manifestations can be just as disabling, and organic/anatomic, as dementia and Down's Syndrome.

Mr. Spears—decades before he left Boston Medical Center against medical advice with his bag of meat in hand—suffered from the complex neuroanatomic damage of horrific, unimaginable childhood trauma. The consequences and effects of this trauma prevented his safe functioning in society. He was too busy reacting and surviving to fully comprehend how to navigate his world—and likely lacked the prefrontal cortex capabilities to do so. He couldn't hold down a job, pay bills, follow through with tasks, or do the hundreds of things each day needed to just function in life. He couldn't even negotiate the relative risks and benefits of prioritizing a bag of rotting meat over effective management of a potentially life-threatening medical condition as he reactively screamed offensive expletives at nervous medical residents in the hospital.

As our knowledge continues to grow and evolve, we can continue to have discussions, hopefully more than arguments, about the extent to which a person's neuroanatomic pathology associated with chronic mental illness and historic trauma requires societal assistance to be safe, successful, and less costly over time. However this debate must be as evidence-based and scientifically informed as possible. If it's not, then we're just guessing. And history has demonstrated we're not that good at guessing; we're usually distracted into wrong directions by convenient, preexisting stereotypes and misconceptions that justify the easy—not necessarily the correct—answers.

Misconceptions are harmful and, increasingly in our society, manipulated, or even intentionally created, by those looking to benefit from them. History is full of predictable patterns of leaders sowing the seeds of conflict and hatred to create an atmosphere of chaos that is conducive to using the tools of dehumanization to grab power.

How we perceive, understand, and interact with our world forms the foundation of our human existence. Our brains constantly process the information we receive and filter it through our beliefs, shaping who we trust, how we engage with others, and how we behave.

Actual reality is not as important as our *perception* of reality. However, the Achilles's heel of our cognitive filters is that they tend to prioritize confirmation over enlightenment and truth—especially when busy or in times of conflict. Our brains more easily accept that which feels familiar and reinforces our already-held beliefs. They don't like to be challenged and stressed. Therefore, the ability to control and direct the cognitive filters of others has always been a type of Holy Grail for those seeking power, votes, money, or just improved social status.

Recently, politicians and media have used the rapid-fire world of social media to constantly bombard us with chaos and conflict—thereby creating stressed environments conducive to controlling the filters through which we view our world. This chaos facilitates the old and familiar political strategy of forming "in-group" cohesion and loyalty while creating indifference—or increasingly, hatred—toward the "out-group." Ignoring our shared 99.9 percent genetically-identical humanity in the development of the "in-group versus out-group" narratives tricks the mind into turning the humanity of "the other" into falsely perceived "automata," reducing them to the status of inanimate objects or animals.

Over the past few years, I've noticed a growing pattern of negative news stories regarding homeless populations. The language of the articles often parallels the languages of dehumanization used in Dr. Harris and Dr. Fiske's study. "Addicts" are often automatically linked to "homeless," and stories increasingly focus on episodes of violence when they occur. I've seen several news stories referring to individuals experiencing homelessness as "vagrants." A few years ago, a headline referenced a "shocking video" of homeless patients using public transportation trains as places to sleep. I naturally clicked the story to see the video (after, of course, watching a 15-second commercial), since the word "shocking" caught my attention in the title. I was "shocked" to see a video of people who were simply sleeping. They looked peaceful—and exhausted. Nothing disruptive. It was more sad than it was shocking. I'm sure the people in the video were not psyched that they were sleeping on the trains, but at least they felt some level of safety and warmth.

As homelessness predictably grows across the US, in many communities, it's becoming a top concern of voters. A May 2023 survey by the J. Ronald Terwilliger Center for Housing Policy and Morning Consult demonstrated that 46 percent of participants have witnessed worsening homelessness in their communities over the past year. Over half of respondents, 58 percent, believe homelessness is a "very serious problem" nationally. Our current trajectories project that homelessness will continue to grow in our nation. People want to, and need to, better understand chronic homelessness—including its complexities and those who suffer from them.

However, the conversations around this worsening social dilemma are quickly becoming, or have already become, wrapped up in this modern political debate climate of us-versus-them—pick a side and hunker down to prove you're right. The vernacular of dehumanization in many of these debates seems to be increasingly intentional—manipulating and "neurohacking" us into division and conflict. And again, this will inevitably result in reaction instead of the collaborative cognition needed to solve the challenging social issue of homelessness *as an actual community*—one that could be, and at its core truly *should* be, united by our common, shared ideals of altruism and "loving thy neighbor."

Any large-scale, political and/or media-pushed dehumanization of people experiencing homelessness will only worsen existing prejudices and predispositions toward misunderstanding. The consequences will be increasingly expensive and dangerous as the homeless crisis in America continues to grow.

Not everything has to be turned into a political debate. In that ever-shrinking Venn-diagram overlap of political party beliefs, there remains some things that are so intuitive and logical that even those more focused on political disagreement than societal improvement can agree upon them.

Tolerating the high societal cost of suffering for our most vulnerable chronically homeless residents, often to the tune of well over six figures annually per individual, is simply an ill-informed waste of taxpayer money. The homeless population is very much part of that top one percent of the population whose medical expenses account for 25 percent, or over one trillion dollars, of our nation's annual medical spend.

How we manage, or mismanage, this top one percent impacts the funding and resources we can spend in other vital social sectors. If we stop and think, common-sense approaches for better managing the underlying causes of chronic homelessness should overlap in the Venn diagram of political agreement—at least to a much larger extent than it currently does.

Clear historic precedence exists for bipartisan solutions around chronic homelessness that work to reduce its high cost. George W. Bush and his administration made tremendous strides by expanding Housing First initiatives that had started more than a decade before he took office. His rationale was as financial as it was humane: Do not wait until people stabilize from a mental, physical, or social health perspective. Just get them into housing, and this will provide a more secure environment to address these typically complex issues that cause us to hemorrhage money in our hospitals, shelters, and jails.

This made sense but was a major shift from historic approaches that required that a person demonstrate stability and control of their issues prior to receiving housing. For many who suffered from chronic homelessness in the context of severe, chronic diseases, this wasn't realistic. This was like asking a diabetic to first demonstrate control of their blood sugars prior to giving them insulin. Housing is healthcare. Lack of housing is a pathology itself that exacerbates other pathologies.

So George W. Bush's administration flipped the thinking by facilitating the widespread adoption of the early Housing First pilots that preceded his administration. The model prioritized getting individuals into housing, messy pathologies and all, as a first step. Intuitively, a more secure social situation—out of the elements, stress, and chaos of homelessness—should facilitate better environments for healing very complex and challenging conditions. This was a significant step in recognizing the urgency of housing and an acknowledgment that, for many, housing should be seen as a prerequisite to improved health—not a reward for obtaining it.

Housing First was successful and offered a major fundamental shift in how politics viewed homelessness. Between 2005 and 2008, it resulted in a 30 percent reduction in homelessness and was ultimately continued in the Obama administration. It was humanistic. It was cost-effective. A study in the medical journal *JAMA* in 2009 demonstrated an impressive societal cost savings of approximately $2,500 monthly for people who participated in such models compared to those who did not—after the cost of housing.[1] People who were housed were not in the expensive safety nets of hospital beds, ambulances, jails, and homeless shelters.

The historic Housing First models exemplify the importance of not reflexively tossing everything into the worsening "pick sides; I am right, you are wrong" political debates in our society. We must remember and recognize the intuitive, powerful nature of political collaboration and cooperation. It's process design. It's problem-solving. It's working smarter, which will mean more collaboratively.

Blind partisanship is its own pathology. It always has been. It's just been becoming more malignant recently.

That Venn diagram overlap of the political beliefs of the left and the right must not shrink to zero. If it does, that's simply forced and manipulated polarization—disagreeing for the sake of disagreeing—which is a ridiculous way to run a country.

If homelessness is increasingly dragged into polarized political dialogue, we'll continue to slowly lose our ability to collaborate across social sectors and governments to solve the expensive, complicated problem involving the suffering of our most vulnerable residents. The easy out of criminalizing homelessness to avoid the intellectually challenging work of solving it will become increasingly tempting—positioning those experiencing it as "the other" and then discarding them through stereotypes and blame. However, untreated pathology, no matter how much you try to ignore it, doesn't go away. It will continue to grow and metastasize into a more advanced, severe, and expensive state.

Improving issues around both new and chronic homelessness will require politicians to collaborate and use their collective cognition to find efficient solutions for the communities they serve. Innovative affordable housing options sit on one end, with improved mental and physical health care, justice reform, and supportive housing on the other. Ideally, these solutions would leverage our often under-recognized, shared social ideals. It will require compromise; if we insist on agreeing on everything before we sit down to discuss anything, we will accomplish nothing. A prerequisite to any effective, long-term solutions, no matter what they may be, is a conducive environment in which to make them.

We can't lose control of the narrative around homelessness, about its realities and the people impacted by it. There's an urgency for us to come together and problem-solve as a community. There are lives, and billions of dollars in taxpayer money, at stake.

―――

As we wait for society and those who run it to get back on track, the first step for us individually might be to fight to stay in control of our own cognitive filters in ways that are consistent with our internal personal values.

Granted, controlling these filters seems to be getting harder, as we all are increasingly exposed to the extremes of the political spectrum. It feels like, more and more, people simply look to their party line, or their favorite media site, to form opinions about whatever topic is being discussed. Instead of analyzing its complexities, increasingly we are reflexively adopting whatever stance we're instructed to.

Those polarizing and manufacturing chaos and conflict aren't working for your own good or interest, or that of society's—but for their own. They're working to consolidate power, or likes, or votes, or income or whatever it is. They want to polarize you into being unable to appreciate, comprehend, or even consider any opinions that differ from yours. They then circle back and reinforce these polarized views with dopamine hits that confirm such manufactured bias and its associated anger. Each side is screaming—trying to draw attention to what the other side is doing while ignoring, or denying, that they themselves are doing the same exact thing.

As homelessness continues to worsen across the nation, getting caught up in the partisan discourse occurring in the news and in politics, I can't help but think that political views may be creeping into clinical judgment and patient management. We don't practice medicine in a vacuum; we all come in with our own beliefs, views, and prejudices. Homelessness has increasingly moved up on the list of political hot-button topics, which to me is dangerous and scary given our growing numbers.

People who suffer from homelessness, like everybody else, desire to love and be loved. To have deep social bonds. To feel a sense of worth. Any application of a dehumanizing stereotype that tries to convince us otherwise is intentionally deceptive. The intentions of those pushing these narratives must be questioned and challenged.

As society becomes more polarized and confusing, going back to our roots, for many of us, may be the key—especially those roots that, for the majority of us, provided an early foundation for the ethics and virtues we strive for. As we go back to our roots with a new, or perhaps renewed, perspective, we may find ourselves having a better understanding of some of the familiar stories and lessons we find there.

As Aristotle and other philosophers and religious leaders throughout history have attempted to teach us, we can also find happiness.

31

UNDER GOD

We often drift through life interacting with the superficialities of others, not with who they truly are at their core.

Mike had an old, worn prayer card with a picture of Jesus on it. Each morning, he would wake up at 4 a.m., typically uncomfortable from a night of sleeping upright in his crowded, broken-down Chevy, which he had parked in the back corner of a parking lot behind a local Olive Garden. He would then pray—for exactly 30 minutes—with his gaze fixed on the prayer card. Afterwards, he would turn on NPR radio and listen for the next two or three hours.

He loved NPR. Almost every conversation I had with him would start with a reference to some story he had heard that morning on the radio. Whether it was conversations on shipping trade routes in Asia or on whether using chalk on tires for parking enforcement was constitutional, he was always excited to discuss the topic and offer his opinions, which were typically very insightful. In fact, I actually started to listen to NPR on my morning driving in to work on the days I was to meet with him, just so I didn't feel lost in our conversations.

I didn't know about the prayer card, however, or his morning prayer routine until two weeks before his death.

I followed Mike for over a year after our homeless outreach team had engaged with him in the parking lot. Another one of our patients had asked that they try to engage with him, concerned about his poor health.

In his early 50s, Mike had been homeless for the past five years after progressive arthritis and cardiac conditions forced him to stop working as a cook—a "damn good one," as he would remind me. He had diffuse arthritis with severe pain in his legs and back. Years earlier, he had gone to a pain clinic and was on numerous pain medications, which took him over a year to taper from after he discovered "nothing really worked." So he lived in pain and never once asked for pain medications—adamantly refusing anything, even Tylenol, when offered.

He also often struggled to breathe. He had a history of several heart attacks. He had a total of three stents placed in his cardiac arteries to keep his vessels open. The damage done to his heart was severe. In September 2018, an echocardiogram demonstrated an ejection fraction—the percent of blood that was ejected with each heartbeat—of less than 25 percent. Normal is 50 to 70 percent. He was diligent about taking his cardiac medications, never missing a dose.

He could no longer work. Even panhandling a few blocks from his car was exhausting. He would have to take a break every block in his daily commute, and he brought a crate so he could sit when he got there.

His legs were often "swollen like tree trunks" due to the synergistic harm of a poorly functioning heart and the effects of gravity from sleeping upright in his car at night. However, he would not—or as he would argue, *could not*—stay in the shelters, no matter how cold, hot, or uncomfortable his car could become or how bad his legs got. He admitted he became too nervous around a lot of people. He preferred to live in his older-model Chevy, painful tree-trunk legs and all, rather than stay in shelters.

He would not typically come to the clinic to see me. So I usually had to go visit him in the parking lot behind Olive Garden. I would often bring dinner from Alpaca—a Peruvian chicken place he loved that he got me hooked on.

Every conversation Mike had was animated. He loved music and would act incredulous when I told him I didn't recognize one of the old time musicians he brought up. "How have you never heard of ...?!" One night, he made me listen to Jimmy Smith's live version of "Root Down" seven times as we ate dinner, each time getting more excited than the last.

He also loved the animals around his car—the squirrels, birds, even the worms. They were his pets. He was particularly fond of a specific family of squirrels. Our conversations would often be interrupted when he saw them. He would then start to talk to them, often spending time to feed them—never in a rush to get back to our conversation.

One night when I stopped by to visit him on my way home from work, he told me about how, that morning, his favorite squirrel had sat on his window and just stared in at him "during my prayer session."

I thought I had known everything about him at this point. Surprised, I asked, "A prayer session?"

"Yeah, every morning I wake up at 4 a.m. and pray. How did you not know that?! It's a major part of who I am." He then showed me his prayer card. "I'm pretty sure He listens."

A few weeks later, we would find Mike deceased in a hotel room that he had agreed to stay in during a heat wave. Just a few months earlier, we had finally gotten him disability and Social Security. He was weeks away from housing at the time of his untimely death. We were so close.

There are so many things I will remember about Mike—his energy, his intellect, his deep spirituality—but the main thing I will remember is his laugh. He had absolutely the best laugh—deep, boisterous, and genuine, defiantly lighting up the darkness he lived in, and in hindsight, perhaps reflecting the "major part" of who he was.

So many of us suffer more in our imaginations than in actual reality. We focus on the few bad things in our lives instead of the abundant good things. We forget gratitude.

Mike flipped this. He saw beauty and hope all around him. He was thankful for what he had, even if it was just broken-down cars, friendly squirrels, occasional Peruvian chicken dinners, or NPR radio. Every day, he worked to perceive his world with optimism and was determined to find the beauty in it, starting every day with his 4 a.m. prayer routine.

―――

Almost three out of four people in the US report that religion is important in their lives, including the 69 percent who are Christian.[1]

The history of humanity is marked by constant tension between selfish human instincts and the beauty of human potential—the easy and reflexive versus the cognitive and inspiring. Religion has served as an inspiration for the latter, yet too often, a demonstration of the former.

History is full of examples of people with spiritual beliefs across the pluralism of our world religions, acting selfishly against those beliefs, hypocritically demonstrating the very instinctual weaknesses their religions were cautioning them about—displaying the worst of humanity instead of fighting for its best. This pattern has driven so many conflicts, wars, and hatred over time. It can be seen in how modern-day followers of religions based on love and altruism are easily distracted, angered, and polarized against others.

These clear patterns of hypocrisy result in supposedly very religious people not necessarily treating others in very religious ways, selectively choosing which teachings they actually want to loudly live out as they silently violate the others. Selfishly twisting religions in self-serving ways. Using religion as a cover for our human flaws instead of an inspiration to address them.

The calls to love others—to embody altruism—are clear and foundational to the world religions that the vast majority of humans follow. However, we have already reviewed the work of Dr. Harris that demonstrates why this can be such a challenge.

The very teaching of unselfish love and putting others before ourselves—"the first shall be last and the last shall be first" (Matthew 20:16)—runs contrary to the human instincts of social hierarchy dominance. In this way, it serves as a warning against the associated predisposed, inhumane, unjust ways we interact with people on both ends of the social hierarchy spectrum—to tolerate, and therefore reward, immorality and deceit at the top while accepting suffering and even directed atrocities against those on the bottom.

These predispositions are perhaps baked into our zero-sum, optimize-resources, survival-of-the-fittest instinctual tendencies that have driven human evolution. However, they blatantly run contrary to the teachings of altruism, fairness, and love preached in religion. Or, even aside from religion, a humanity itself that has undergone rapid—perhaps even exponential—cognitive and, consequently, social changes over the past few thousand years.

I would like to think we have changed for the better in many ways. The genetic and instinctual hardwiring of our bodies and minds, however, slowly adapts and evolves through one generational, random genetic mutation at a time. And this process hasn't necessarily kept up with our cognitive, frontal-lobe-mediated social evolution. Instincts of survival, social hierarchy placement, and dehumanization have, in many ways, become somewhat maladaptive evolutionary relics. They haven't evolved quickly enough to keep pace with the altruism increasingly striven for in the philosophy, religion, and teachings of our society.

It's clear that the human brain, through awareness and understanding, can work to intentionally override instincts. The uniquely strong cognitive abilities of the human brain ensure we're not captive to the neurobiological instincts of the more "reactive" parts of our brain, which prioritize survival and the maximizing our own personal comfort. In many ways, this seems to be the basis of so many religious teachings which, at their core, involve overcoming selfish human instincts to look outward and make the world a better place. It's the one thing that makes the human brain completely badass and unparalleled to other species. In many ways, these cognitive abilities define the uniqueness of our humanity and are foundational to faith.

We can do hard things, placing short-term pain/discomfort into the perspective of long-term gains and benefits. The evolving science of neurobiology is increasingly demonstrating just how beneficial it is for us to do hard things that are good for us. Exercising, studying, overcoming addiction, making ourselves stand in a really cold shower, or—what can be the hardest of all of these—unselfishly looking outward to help, listen to, and love others.

Empathy is believed to lie in the insula and anterior cingulate cortex parts of the human brain.[2] These parts also involve tenacity and persistence. Being tenacious and persistent when challenged, especially with something really hard or unpleasant, has been shown not only to improve academic and job success, but health as well.[3] When we do hard things, this part of the brain grows.

There's a reason why people who look outward and practice empathy are healthier and live longer. Remaining in a state of hate, resentment, and manipulated polarization could very well be the equivalent of sitting on the couch all day, eating junk food and playing video games. Doing so may be convenient and easy at the time, but ultimately it is unhealthy.

Religions developed during a time when nobody could imagine that we would discover the intricacies of how our minds work. But we have—or at least we have started to. Obviously if historical religious leaders in their time had preached to "use the cognitive function of your prefrontal cortex to override the evolutionary-based, social-hierarchy related instincts," they would have lost their audiences. But so much of their focus on altruism goes directly to this idea. The neurobiology of altruism often has a battle on its hands with human instinct. Yet historic religious teachings were so often directed at how we can work, think, and act to be successful.

Individually, to live a life of determined and cognitive love can allow us to live longer and better (the two major goals of medicine)—and, many believe, when our time on earth is over, improve our chances of getting a fast-pass at the pearly gates. (I don't think anybody believes, "How well do you hate and dehumanize?" will be a question on the entrance exam.)

In the context of the science of social cognition and associated neuroanatomy, there is a potential to evolve religious beliefs to get closer to their ultimate goals around altruism and love of others.

Most of us, such as the soccer dad disgruntled by his son's team placement, are likely aware of the hypocrisies of our actions relative to our professed beliefs. Yet the tendencies around dehumanization and selfish social hierarchy placement are strong enough to sustain these hypocrisies despite the internal religious beliefs we strive to live up to. If we can better understand these mechanisms—including why we are predisposed to these hypocrisies—and recognize them in ourselves when they occur, it may empower us on the individual level to better live up to these ideals that we desperately seek to practice.

Admittedly, this often feels like it's almost impossible. It's hard to see "God in others" when we reflexively see the "others" in others. As we learn the reasons why it's so difficult, we also learn why it's actually not impossible—and why it's so important.

Instead of reflexively "conflict resolution-ing" dehumanization, per Dr. Harris's research, we must use the ability we all have to think and override it. We all can do so. Perhaps we will all one day be reminded about this when we're at those pearly gates. If we better understand the mechanism of instincts and selfishly motivated reflexives, we can also better follow Blu's plea to stop, think, and just listen openly to one another. That is the door to humanization.

If we do this, I think we will be surprised by what we find.

During my career, I've seen a lot of downstream manifestations of trauma, insecurity, and fear. I've seen reactions. I've seen a lot of incredibly complex pathologies that ravage patients and shape their interaction with the world—complexities impossible to appreciate simply through common daily interactions. But I have not seen much intrinsic "badness." I think inherent goodness and beauty in humanity are much more common than we believe. This is an objective observation, not naïve blindness—at least I think it is.

Fortunately we do not necessarily need to, especially on an individual interaction level, figure it all out. As we are taught, our job is not to judge others; it's to love others.

Look hard for the good in others. If you can't find it, look harder. It's there—almost always—and most religions call for us to find it.

Altruism indeed can have its own selfish motivations. Being nice and compassionate has been associated with greater health and sense of well-being,[4] providing scientific evidence to Dalai Lama's famous quote, "If you want *others* to be happy, practice compassion. If *you* want to be happy, practice compassion." This echo's Aristotle's teaching from thousands of years earlier. He had no idea what the prefrontal cortex was, but he knew of its importance. "Life is a gift of nature, but beautiful living is the gift of wisdom. … It's the active exercise of our faculties in conformity with virtue that causes happiness, and the opposite activities its opposite." For Aristotle, virtue involved practicing both kindness and compassion.[5]

Spending our days trying to climb over others in the pursuit of social dominance can be draining. Seeking the validation of others often proves futile. There is no end goal; it's not really attainable. Rarely will people offer you the praise, validation, and social status you desire; they're often too busy climbing the same social hierarchy ladder, trying to step over you in the process.

In contrast, there is potential instant-feedback gratification in the love of others—in altruism—that not only makes others around you happier, but you as well. It's a much easier way to release social-interaction-related dopamine, serotonin, and oxytocin hits compared to desperate attempts at dominance. The impact of love and altruism is something attainable that you can easily appreciate daily—by choosing to act on it.

Deep down, if we have enough confidence and security in ourselves, perhaps supported by the foundational religious ideals most people believe in, we don't need to participate in the relatively futile and exhausting game of optimizing social dominance and hierarchy. Perhaps the best way to "win" the daily game of social hierarchy placement is to not play it at all.

In the end, none of us will escape Banksy's second death. Immortality is not achievable. Status, reputation, and immortality are all fool's gold. Some might be able to avoid it longer than others, but ultimately all of us will be forgotten from this world. Which, as world religions remind us, is okay; it's not about that. What is attainable is how we can live up to our uniquely human potential while on this Earth—through love, kindness, and cognition.

The science of social cognition and associated altruism doesn't need religion to support it, yet it intuitively does. Conversely, this is a case where science can support the underlying ideals and beliefs of religion, not refute them. It can provide context to understand both the teaching of world religions as well as their flawed human applications throughout history. Our historic failures to live up to ideals of altruism, and love should not be misinterpreted as evidence against their validity or possibilities.

I will back out of this religious tangential, as I imagine this is like watching a minister, imam, rabbi, or priest trying to diagnose pancreatitis. The simple point is this: If people *actually* practiced the altruism preached so loudly across the plurality of religions, our world would be a much kinder, happier, healthier, and efficient place.

Opportunities exist in the daily interactions we all have with others. These opportunities are constant—in how we interact with family, friends, strangers, and those suffering the most in our communities. We can work on changing our focus on self toward focus on others. Perhaps we can practice Jim O'Connell's "pre-admiration," as we enter social interactions—appreciating the potential good in people even before we actually know them. To follow Blu's example of love and humanization instead of the opposite.

There was a desperation in Blu's advocacy, as she knew firsthand the nightmares of homelessness, trauma, and addiction. Blu is no longer with us, but her message can be. She was pleading for society to pay attention. To listen to those who were experiencing homelessness. Truly listen so as to better understand. Better understand so as to better love. This would ultimately allow us to gain perspective, so we can better follow Fr. Greg Boyle's (fellow Loyola High School grad!) advice in his book, *Tattoos of the Heart*: to develop "a compassion that can stand in awe at what the poor have to carry rather than stand in judgment at how they carry it." That is love—foundational to the ideals of religions.

Coincidentally, it's also an awesome public health strategy.

Besides, seeing the beauty and joy of others is a much more pleasant way to live than reflexively seeing their flaws. And ultimately, this much more accurate assessment of the reality around us can help pull us out of the thinly veiled hypocrisies in which we often live.

This mindset will be essential if we are to be both humanistic, and therefore efficient, in how we address the growing complexities of homelessness in our society.

32

BREAK ZONE

As a kid growing up in Los Angeles, I loved going to the beach. I found just sitting on the beach or playing in the sand boring. I had to be in the water. I would run out into the waves right when we arrived, staying in the water for hours and often being a bit too brave/stupid.

Waves along Southern California beaches can get big, especially from the perspective of a young kid. I would go out with my siblings or friends and spend the day bodysurfing, boogie boarding, or later in my childhood, surfing. Sometimes, I would just go in alone. The goal was always to get to where the waves perfectly peaked and curled down the line without breaking directly on top of you. To get there, however, you had to get through the "break zone." Even experienced surfers will occasionally get caught in the break zone. As a kid, I would frequently get demolished there.

The waves traveled thousands of miles before starting to break on the seabed. I would often get stuck meeting them just a few seconds too late. When the waves got big, this could be scary. I could see a wave coming right at me, starting to break, and know there was nothing I could do to prevent it from crashing right on top of me. Often, the wave would push me down, thrashing me around and holding me underwater for a short time, although it could feel like an eternity. When I finally got control, I would pop back up above the water and catch my breath, often only to find another wave about to crash on top of me. When the waves came in sets, this could result in a cycle of ass-kickings which, in hindsight, were probably very entertaining for any surfers or fellow beachgoers who may have been watching. But, all it took was catching one wave and riding it in, and it all became worth it—even if, right after, I found myself once again in that same break zone.

As I grew older, I learned to stay calmer in the break zone. Instead of being scared, resisting and fighting when a wave was pushing me under, I would try to relax, knowing from experience that things would be OK. If I could wait it out, the thrashing wave would pass, things would calm down, and I could get back up. I learned to appreciate, even enjoy, the chaos in the break zone. A simple and deliberate change of perspective could change the scary into the challenging and rewarding.

I've had to adopt the same mindset over the years to adjust to the constant waves of evolving chaos in medicine and their impact on homeless populations—whether that be pandemics, ever-changing social and housing initiatives, depleted community resources, or the changing whims and moving goalpost of medical payers. In public health, these waves can often feel like tsunamis. We approach the challenges knowing our interventions will never be enough—not good enough, not large enough, and not urgent enough. We go in knowing there will often be resistance, and even resentment, from an American healthcare system that has historically been both deliberate and strategic in its efforts to avoid this chaos outside of its medical walls. We know we will often get it wrong. We know we will get pushed down and thrown around by the chaos. It's inevitable.

As we continue to work in the break zones of medicine, however, we can draw inspiration from the determined resilience of the patients we find there with us, trying their best to survive and keep their heads above water through the constant onslaught of waves crashing on them. Their efforts were epitomized in a quote from Peter in response to my encouragement not to give up—to keep trying—prior to me leaving Boston. "Of course I'm going to try. What other option do I have?" Life is much easier when we don't confuse ourselves with options that do not, or should not, exist. Ultimately, the vocation of medicine mandates we have no choice *but* to be there in the chaos of the break zone with our patients, as they have no choice but to be there themselves.

What other option do we have? We simply cannot tolerate the expensive and avoidable suffering of vulnerable patients. It's inhumane, anti-vocational, and increasingly a horrifically expensive public health strategy to do so.

But how do we build strategies to sustain and survive in the break zone? When working in the chaos, it's natural to develop a sense of desperation and associated burnout as we witness the suffering of the patients we're struggling to care for. The individuals who are desperate, even panicked, as they reach out for help that, ultimately, we often can't provide. The lives we can't save and the suffering we can't efficiently address. There is so much loss in the break zone. Not only of health and life, but also of beauty and goodness and the potential that often has gone largely unnoticed by the world—despite it being obvious even through simple human interactions. The world just never tried to look for it.

The memories of those we lost can be haunting ... but they can also inspire us to do better.

Part of the long-term strategy around sustaining work in public health may be redefining success so as to better recognize it when present. Success is relative. Success in medicine is not always a cure. In fact, it often is not. We typically don't "cure" diabetes, or heart disease; we "manage" them. Clinical success often means better control—less suffering and less morbidity. Success can be when a life of loneliness doesn't end with dying alone. It can be less pain, less stress, or less isolation. It can be a person better understanding their history, their body, or their previously unrecognized personal strength of resilience. It can be people finally getting disability benefits, in the context of the qualifying diseases they suffer from, which can then help them not to go hungry or get housing. It can be as simple as validation and humanization—a smile, laugh, or joke—or as amazing and brilliant as overcoming constant social and medical barriers to one day walk up in front of a crowded lecture hall at Harvard Medical School to enlighten future doctors and inspire them to right our historic wrongs … and not be "shitheads" as they do so.

As we continue to advocate for larger system changes, better recognizing these often-subtle successes in our patients can help to sustain our efforts. We can gain some reassurance that as our patients continue to suffer expensively and die early, at least they were not alone. We worked with them. Listened. Humanized. Saw their beauty. Alleviated their suffering, even if just a little.

We can, and it's important that we do, take this consolation.

But not too much.

For the truth is that, ultimately, it is a relatively weak justification that we need to make sure we balance. Patients were not looking *just* for support. Or pity. Or a friend. They were definitely not looking for enablement. They were looking for an end to their suffering from their poorly understood pathologies. They were desperately seeking help to not drown, not simply for comfort as they did so. They were looking for any help they could get in their determined and impossible fight to extract resilience out of absolutely nothing.

For so many, we were not able to provide that for them. We were often not even close. That can be such a painful and brutal reality to deal with.

We must work to ensure that our ignorance, and our associated discomfort, don't predispose us to possibly seek too much reassurance in a "comfort care" mindset—prioritizing patient comfort instead of an aggressive push toward cure. We start to rationalize. We can become complacent with less sense of urgency. In this state of complacency, we can start to facilitate, even enable, disease progression instead of continuing to fight it.

Enablement, if we're not careful, can simply be the other side of the same coin as neglect. In our field, both, no matter how well rationalized, are deadly. Both make the intense and uncomfortable suffering of those we're engaging with more tolerable *for us*—providing blinders that we utilize to stay functional.

And, I would argue, both are dehumanizing.

Ideally, safety nets should empower patients to improve their health, not trap them in their pathologies. They should save patients from dangerous symptoms while effectively identifying and treating root causes.

For ultimately, any consolation that there was "nothing we could really do" is, from a physiologic perspective, fundamentally inaccurate. Pathology, once its mechanisms and pathways are known, can almost always be altered. If we know how something works, we can figure out how to stop it by disrupting or changing how it functions.

There's just so much we don't know about how mental health, trauma, stress, and social determinants impact the body. Community-based, beyond our control, these social pathologies have proven to be much more complicated and confusing than those pathologies we study in controlled labs. So we often give up in frustration, stop trying to improve, and collapse back into the broken but comfortable … and reimbursed. We continue to watch as patients suffer and die expensively in front of us, often using our instinctual crutches of dehumanization and anterior cingulate cortex mediated conflict resolution to rationalize and move on. We shoulder-shrug incredible people with incredible strength and resilience into early graves as we convince ourselves there was nothing we could do to help.

Dr. Craik must have been haunted as he watched his longtime friend, patient, and president slowly asphyxiate in front of him. He had to have known he was off in his "balanced humor approach" and associated therapeutic "bleed out" attempts—that there was some underlying cause he was missing as a physician.

We can't get comfortable in a palliative mindset. We must always continue to push for cure. Always.

All that genius, determination, and innovation we demonstrate chasing our fee-for-service financial goals must be applied, times two, to pathologies that are much more nebulous and complex than ones we can control in our clinical silos. As they challenge our competency, highlight our current ignorance, and agitate our ego, we will need humility which, historically, hasn't been our strength in medicine.

It's true that our patients were looking to not drown, not for comfort as they did so. It is also true that providing that comfort, companionship, and humanization in our efforts, while infinitely insufficient, was infinitely better than doing nothing. And therein lies the paradox that makes providing care for individuals experiencing homelessness the most uplifting, depressing, energizing, exhausting, inspirational, and deflating job in healthcare—and, without a doubt, the most rewarding. We have to continue to evolve and appreciate that all our efforts, both successful and unsuccessful, should ultimately advance us from our current, often blood-letting-ish state toward the progress we are fighting for—both at an individual and a population level.

(See Appendix 4: Righting our Historic Wrongs: The Potential for Medical Education to Help Evolve Us Closer to Vocational Efficiency).

In the fall of 2022, we opened WakeMed's Center For Community Health, Innovation, and Equity. In this trauma-informed collaborative care model, medical and behavioral health providers, under the same roof, work to stabilize the health of our community's highest-risk and most vulnerable patients. Once stabilized, our patients are "graduated" into one of our community partner's medical and behavioral health clinics for long-term management. We share notes, make calls, or even have joint visits as we do these "warm hand-offs" with our community partners—working as a team. We help to pass on not only patient information, but also clinical trust that can be leveraged into establishing long-term relationships as we move on to help the next people falling into our safety net.

The clinic itself is beautiful, with its trauma-informed design and architecture meticulously mapped out by Dr. Nerissa Price. The medical exam rooms are adjacent to our trauma therapists' and behavioral health care managers' offices. All patients are screened for depression and anxiety when they come into the clinic. Psychiatry will see patients when medical providers feel like it's necessary, or just provide quick advice on the medical providers' clinical questions. Our case managers will often come in for visits with the patients and work with them to address their social issues. Housing agencies and community providers can connect with our patients there. One of our best-received interventions is our spiritual care chaplain, Tina Morris-Anderson, who will meet with interested patients in the meditation room off our front lobby. We also have a large room where we offer "Seeking Safety" trauma group therapy. In this same room, we assemble every quarter with our community advisory board, a group of local, faith-based community and government leaders who provide vital input to help guide our community health outreach and educational efforts.

We put a whiteboard in every room. During visits with patients, I am often up at the board explaining and teaching "mechanism"—educating through my admittedly horrific artistic renditions of how the body and mind work (or do *not* work). This often involves changing the conversation from "what the hell is wrong with me?" to "this is what is happening to me." Dr. Price has a favorite saying that sums up the work we do at the center: "We need to share our secrets with our patients instead of holding on to them tightly." Our main secret: *Medicine is often really not that complicated—especially when we start to understand mechanism.* We just need to do a better job making sure our patients understand what they are battling.

And in the front lobby ... two more whiteboards with the "joke of the week" written on them, one in English and one in Spanish. (We have processes in place to ensure they're always hilarious.) A brain engaged in humor may be a little less engaged with stress.

The model has received increased attention recently; we have had visits from local political leaders, hospital CEOs from across the nation, the State Department for our Hostage US work, and the White House itself. Yet it is still often ineffective. Too often, we're still not able to save patients from poor outcomes and mortality. Patients still drown. It's still haunting. But it feels like it is happening less. We still get our asses kicked by pathology on a daily basis, but at least we're better understanding root causes as we continue to try to attack them as a team. And on occasion, we are starting to see "miracles" with some of our more impossible cases.

In our first year, the center scored in the top 1 percent of PRC scores, which measure patient satisfaction and experience. Since we care for patients who often struggle with distrust, given their historic negative experiences with healthcare systems, we found this important—and hopeful.

It feels like we're on the right track, finally tackling root causes instead of chasing symptoms. It's far from perfect or even good—but it's better. At the very least, it feels like the expensive bloodletting is beginning to stop.

The cost savings with many of our patients goes easily into the six figures. Sometimes you have to prove the intuitive, and it feels like we are—that one of the most cost-effective approaches in the evolving world of value-based care might simply be erasing the hypocritical gaps between our vocational roots and our actual patient care.

PART VI
LOVE

33

IN THE END

Over the years, Joanne Guarino and I have routinely kept in touch with a phone call every few weeks or so. The calls are usually when I'm driving home from work or shuttling kids around at night. In the earlier years, I admit I kept these calls off speakerphone to prevent having to explain some new words to my young kids. Later, I just became too lazy, and my kids became too excited to listen and talk to her. She cracked them up. After the calls, I sometimes would explain what these new words meant and why they can't use them, but why Miss Joanne could. My youngest son somehow got access to my phone one day and changed the picture that pops up when she calls to a sign simply stating, "The Legend." As a dad, exposing my kids to her personality, wisdom, and general approach to life has been awesome. Over the years, they started to pick up on her catchphrase—"love ya"—to me, to them, and often to the numerous people she was talking to in the background while on the phone.

In 2018, a group of city officials and local leaders from Raleigh and Wake County went to Boston as part of their annual tradition of visiting other cities to study and assess best practices. During the visit, I coordinated a tour of the BHCHP's respite care center, wanting the group to see the facility in hopes we could duplicate the model to some extent in Raleigh. Barry Bock, their incredible CEO at the time, and Jim O'Connell were gracious enough to facilitate the visit. Joanne agreed to help lead the tour.

She was in her usual form—articulate, spontaneous, and hilarious as she effortlessly made the benefits of respite seem intuitive, all while dishing out the "love ya's" to both the staff and patients we bumped into along the way. She had no issues stopping the larger tour group to talk to them—unrushed and personal.

One evening, I called her as she was ending a community advisory board meeting. I insisted that I call her back after she was done. She insisted that I stay on the line … and then insisted that I shut up after I tried to push back. So I shut up. My son and I cracked up hearing her say goodbye to everybody as they left this meeting. It was a parade of one "love ya" after another to her fellow community board members.

A small act, almost habit, serving as an important testament to the potential and beauty of humanity. After all the years of struggles and battles, it represents a resilient and defiant middle finger to the historical trauma that worked so hard to darken her world. She says it so naturally. It's amazing how therapeutic a "love ya" can be, especially when dished out as authentically as she does—almost casually, and definitely not caring if it breaks any social norms. Joanne is all about breaking social norms, especially if they're dumb. She seemingly found the antidote to the darkness and hate of trauma, and made it seem simple. Confident and unapologetic, with "love ya's," because, well, "fuck it"—why not?

Paul was part of the old-school crowd who lived mainly around Boston Common. He had been a beloved patient of BHCHP's Street Team for years. He rarely used shelters, even when it was cold. Like so many of our patients, his worldly experiences and struggles appeared to have afforded him hard-won knowledge of the world around him that he occasionally would share with others. He was quiet but typically smiling and pleasant-mannered.

Paul was admitted to our respite care facility after struggling with symptoms of fatigue and weight loss. His intake labs showed a significant new iron deficiency anemia. Between this and his history of constipation and intermittently seeing blood in his stool, it was not long before our suspicions of colon cancer were confirmed. At the time of diagnosis, it was already widely metastasized. He was in his early 60s.

Receiving news of metastatic, and likely terminal, cancer is difficult for anybody—especially when one lacks strong social support and is experiencing homelessness. Paul initially tried to handle it stoically—at least externally. He asked all the right questions about treatment options and what to expect. After one long discussion with his oncology doctors around his prognosis of "less than a few months," his stoic nature did falter a bit. "I wish I could say I can look back at life and say it's without regrets, but unfortunately it's full of them."

Paul had made the request to have his end-of-life care provided at our respite care center.

Over the years, we had worked to make end-of-life care an option at BHCHP's respite care facility. Trusting clinical relationships are everything, especially while navigating the dying process. For many of our chronically homeless patients, the clinical relationships we shared with them were some of the most supportive and strongest that the patients had in their lives. Patients with terminal illnesses felt much more comfortable at our respite facility where they were known, compared to a random nursing home or hospice center. When those were the only options provided for our patients, they would often refuse, with their inevitable and predictable deaths occurring either on the streets or in the chaotic, cold, sterile, and ultimately lonely environment of a local ICU. This was unsettling for the staff. It felt like the ultimate insult—lives that often started in trauma, stress, and loneliness ending there as well.

We'd been working with a palliative care team through Mass General to improve how we clinically facilitated end-of-life care in respite. With their help and guidance, both in terms of overall clinical protocols and on individual patient management when needed, we were able to care for patients with terminal illnesses through to their deaths.

Paul was clear in his desire to die at McInnis House. He saw death coming and was determined to go out on his terms.

And he tried to reconcile some of his regrets that resulted from a lifetime of addiction and homelessness.

He reached out to all his Boston Common friends with whom he had spent years battling the challenges of living on the streets, and had real conversations about the relationships they shared and what they meant to him.

He also contacted a priest he had interacted with a few years back. Paul and his family were very religious growing up. He still identified strongly with his faith despite all the struggles that resulted in a guilt that had pushed him away from practicing it. He felt like practicing his faith was hypocritical given the direction his life had gone in.

I'm not sure if there is any greater dopamine- and/or serotonin-depleting gut punch than feeling ostracized and unworthy of participating in a faith in which you strongly believe—to feel disconnected from God. Indeed, evidence has demonstrated the adverse mental and physical health effects of loss of spirituality and its calming influence on the body and mind.[1] Reconnection to the foundational spirituality of individuals, when possible (and desired by the patient), can be more therapeutic than any medical intervention.

For Paul, it was therapeutic. He felt like a load of guilt he had been carrying around for a lifetime was lifted in his final days. Reconnection to his faith provided reassurance and peace.

Paul also reconnected with family, reaching out to his sister living in the Midwest whom he hadn't seen for decades. A month before his death, she came to Boston to spend a few days with Paul. This was transformative for him.

It was moving to see their closeness as siblings. It was as if they'd never missed a beat. The staff reported their interactions as "very brother and sister-ish," which was relatable for many of us. The visit brought nostalgia for better times as they reminisced about the idealisms of youth they both shared, growing up with just one year difference between them. Before the addiction. Before the struggles. Before the stereotypes. Paul's interactions with his sister reminded him of who he truly was, contrasting with society's false, dehumanizing, and reflexive judgments that he'd internalized over time. His sister returned to her family after a few days but still called frequently to check in.

The empowering glow from that visit never left Paul, even as his cancer, right on cue, relentlessly progressed. He grew weaker.

A few days before his death, when he was still able to speak, Paul remained very much at peace. In one of his more contemplative moments, he talked about how much the last two months had meant to him—the sense of relief they provided. Chronic burdens felt lifted. Though he was increasingly emaciated, he had a strength as he spoke that day that seemed to overpower his rapidly deteriorating physical health.

As we ended the conversation, he said something that I've reflected back on constantly since. In a quiet voice through dried and cracked lips, his tone completely at peace, he reflected, "I've been reminded that Love is greater than hate. Good is stronger than bad. And, in the end, I think that is all that really matters."

Given the doses of hatred and "badness" he'd been exposed to, I found this testimony particularly powerful.

In the days that followed, Paul stopped eating and drinking. He eventually stopped communicating. We kept him comfortable. A staff member was constantly by his side, watching over him. While time of death is difficult to anticipate or predict, one evening a nurse called me at home to report a weakening pulse and his breaths being interrupted by gasps, which made me feel like his passing was imminent. I'd agreed to try to be there when things progressed, as sometimes very predictable, typical end-of-life symptoms can rattle and bother staff who aren't familiar with them.

That night, we kept Paul comfortable and sat by his bedside. We had arranged a single room for him. Outside his window, you could see the lights and traffic of the streets of Boston that he had spent so much time on. He was a favorite with the staff who had gotten to know him over the years. As he lay peacefully throughout the evening, he became no longer responsive to any stimuli or communication. Still, a constant flow of staff came in to say their goodbyes —to sit with him and take watch during the night. Some read him poems and stories. Some played soft music or sang. Some prayed with him.

As his breathing became more and more agonal, he paradoxically looked more and more calm.

Around 5 a.m., Paul took his last breath. The room became completely quiet. Outside the window, the streets he'd spent his life on seemed to pause. Completely still. No sounds, no cars … nothing. A few seconds passed before the sounds of sirens and a loud argument broke through the silence. But for a moment, the streets seemed to pay their respects—his peaceful death a well-deserved contrast to the chaotic life he'd experienced on the streets.

I haven't seen many miracles in my career, but there have been a few—things that are hard or even impossible to explain.

I had made a promise to his sister that I would call her when Paul passed away, no matter what time it was. As it was so early in the morning, I started the call by apologizing for waking her up.

"You didn't wake me up. I woke up 12 minutes ago. I knew he was gone. I felt a sense of peace." It was his exact time of death that I had already listed in his notes.

"How did he pass?" she asked.

Thankfully, I was able to respond: "Peacefully … and loved."

34

ONE COGNITIVE THOUGHT

The human brain is vulnerable to instinctual, selfish predispositions that can create significant darkness and suffering for others. Those experiencing homelessness were often traumatically exposed to extremes of this darkness very early, forcing their life trajectories toward pain and hardship.

However, the potential to cognitively override these instincts and pathologies can result in almost unimaginable acts of beauty, love, and altruism.

Look hard, and you will almost always find, even in the worst aspects of our humanity, the light of those challenging—and often overpowering—larger systems of darkness.

In the violence and terror of genocidal hate that Dr. Lasana Harris studied are the Schindlers and Rusesabaginas.

In the painful isolation of homelessness are the Blus and the Joannes.

And in the illness and suffering and death of those neglected by the misaligned priorities of a $4-trillion-dollar healthcare machine, you can find O'Connells and Monroes—and along with them, all the providers, nurses, social workers, case managers, and peer support professionals who work tirelessly to help patients drowning in the chaos of the break zone.

Their examples serve as reminders of the power of human potential—of our boundless capacity to lift one another up. Brilliant displays of determined love and cognition, shining through the darkness that is often hardwired into human instinct, providing hope in the demonstration of the possible.

Brilliant, but often subtle. Brilliant often *because* they are subtle.

Of course, there are also the smaller, more inconspicuous examples all around us—beauty in the humanity of others we completely miss or ignore. If we pause to look for it, we will find it. For me, these subtle displays have provided reassurance and guidance. They've inspired a constant barrage of "aha" moments and continuously challenged my misconceptions and predispositions. Ultimately, they have guided me back to the values and ideals of my childhood; to simple lessons learned as a kid in school, church, and books that I somehow became distracted away from with age.

I've frequently thought back to the message in Paul's last words since his death: *love is greater than hate*. I know his testament was that of a man who reached his conclusion even after experiencing some of the darkest aspects of humanity throughout his lifetime. I instantly recognized his message in the big block letters of Blu's "LOVE WINS" tattoo, in Peter's "I Love Boston" teddy bear key chain that still hangs in my office, in Joanne's "love ya's!" and in Mike's boisterous laugh and worn-out prayer card. It's what wakes up the prefrontal cortexes in the MRIs of Dr. Harris's follow-up studies. It's displayed in the random acts of kindness seen in the homeless community as they look out for one another. It's lived out in the daily, determined humanity of the amazing people I work with in my field of medicine as we all, often blindly, struggle to do our best to keep our heads above water. I find condolence in it when trying to comprehend the senseless acts of violence and evil of humanity that are prioritized in the news over the less interesting displays of love and beauty. I recognize it in church on Sundays, and especially on Easter every year.

Specifically in medicine, we don't just have an obligation to believe Paul's message, we *absolutely* have a vocational obligation to help prove it in our daily work. We can no longer continue to create systems that expensively exacerbate instead of efficiently treat. For as our knowledge advances, ignorance evolves into negligence, opportunities into obligations, and historic inefficiencies into blatant violations of one of the foundations of the Hippocratic Oath: *Do no harm.*

However you look at it, our collective humanity is the summation of all of our individual daily interactions with each other. We have constant opportunities to improve how we interact with those around us. Ultimately, we can only control our own world. Our own cognitive thoughts. Our own actions and how they influence the world for those around us. We can only control our relatively small contribution to the overall sum of humanity. It may be small, but it's tangible.

Even doing "a little" can be infinitely better than nothing, especially if it serves as an example for others. Changing medicine—or the world—may not actually be that hard. It can start with one human interaction at a time—perhaps, as Blu begged us, by choosing to pause, listen, and humanize.

It's a mindset that will be essential if we are to create an environment conducive to the problem-solving that will be needed to live up to our ideals and potential, across our social sectors. A solution for homelessness will not come in one brilliant aha moment, providing a holy-grail-type answer that has been eluding us for years. Solutions will only come through the collaborative application of our collective human cognition, filtered through the lens of our shared ideals. That's how we can work to erase the hypocritical gaps in our society that expensively harm and kill.

I have become increasingly convinced throughout my career that Paul was right about the strength of love. Admittedly, at times I have doubted it. Hate is everywhere. In recent years, it has metastasized throughout the media and through both sides of the political aisle. It can be instinctual. It's easy, especially when dished out through social media. It's almost always a symptom of deep-seated insecurity. It tends to be loud, desperate for attention. Yet its loudness should not be misinterpreted as prevalence ... or strength.

Love often takes more effort and definitely more thought than hate. It also takes more confidence. But ultimately, as Paul reminds us, love overpowers hate. It just does so quietly, with much more humility. Perhaps in our modern world, we just need to be more intentional and much louder in love than those obsessed with hate and polarization. To live our lives looking outward, in love, may also be one of the best things we can do for our health.

We have never understood love, hate, and human interaction like we do today. *Knowledge of mechanism is everything*—including a prerequisite to cure.

The instincts of dehumanization are in each of us. But so is the ability to override them. Ultimately love does, or at least *can*, win ... but only if we intentionally choose to prove it, one human interaction—or, perhaps, one deliberate, cognitive thought—at a time.

ACKNOWLEDGMENTS

I started to write this book early on a random Saturday morning in 2020 when my dog woke me up with her obnoxious barking. Over the following years, it was pieced together on nights, weekends, or any other time I could grab a few minutes. It was a long journey I could have never traveled without my wife, Colleen's, support, encouragement, and understanding. Her belief in me, and more importantly her patience with me, kept me going. Col, I promise I am done writing … for now … I think.

The first person I pulled into this journey outside of Colleen was my brother, Scott—my "original editor"—a brilliant writer whose insights and advice helped to shape this book into something I could be proud of as a first-time author. Trust me; it was not always easy for him. I am grateful for his patience and guidance.

I've been a doctor now for more than 20 years and have become convinced that most of our learning in medicine does not come from textbooks or journals, but from the patients themselves. I've been fortunate to have served uniquely awesome and inspiring patients over the years. Obviously, for confidentiality reasons, I'm not able to thank them by name, but I literally have had thousands of patients, from all different backgrounds and in all different settings, who I have been honored to learn from. You all know who you are—thank you.

A special thank you to everybody at Boston Health Care for the Homeless for their amazing leadership and mentorship: Dr. Jim O'Connell, Dr. Monica Bharel, Dr. Greg Wagoner, Dr Jessie Gaeta, Dr. Thoko Lipato, Dr. Shunda McGahee, Barry Bock, Carolyn

Abbanat, Kathleen Saunders, Dr. Travis Baggett, James Noonan, Rita Chapman, and the rest of their medical providers and staff who taught me so much so early in my career. I will be forever grateful for your examples of humility, brilliance, patience, and love that helped to "sell me" on this extraordinarily awesome, and often brutally challenging, field of medicine—and of course to Joanne Guarino, the best teacher of all time.

Our hotspotter model at WakeMed evolved around the incredible work of our case management team; my knowledge and insights have evolved by watching their work with our patients. I want to acknowledge each one by name, as I recognize that they do not get the appreciation they deserve for the impossible work they do on a daily basis, jumping into the chaos with our patients, right beside them, to help them the best they can. I am constantly inspired and enlightened by their work that provides examples of how medicine *should* work: Jane Smith, Tara Jaworski, Florence Okorie-Mazi, John Harris, Malinda Dunn, Christy Luck, David Combs, Carla MacKenzie, Aurora Dowdy, Cheri Holder, Emily Snipes, Laurie Lassiter, Quiana Battle, Shentelle Livan, Vinett Daley, Keisha Ward, Keturah Beckham, John Garcia Diaz, Kristen Girardi, Donald Baker, Chris Weedy, Theresa Preston, Kris Williford, Gloria Turner, Chris Eldreth, Diana Marroquin-Jimenz, Bobbi Nathan, Connie Lewis, Lwiza Escobar Garcia, Asia Hight, and finally, to Liz Lobaton for keeping all of us organized! Thanks to Marni Cahill, Susan Davis, and Karen Gall for their leadership of this team over the years and, of course, Jen McLucas for building it. I am grateful to have had the opportunity to work with Dr. Arlene Smith and learn from her expertise as she developed our outreach models that evolved over time into more housing opportunities for our patients. It has been an incredible journey.

A special thank you to Dr. Nerissa Price for bringing her experience and leadership to help build our clinical models as well as our community-based outreach efforts.

My entire career has focused on getting out of our medical silos and into the community. I am thankful for all the dedicated leadership in Raleigh and Wake County—which has intentionally built a unique environment of collaboration that has been leveraged into national public health models—including Mayor Mary-Ann Baldwin, Sig Hutchinson, James West, Denise Foreman, Kevin Fitzgerald, Chris Budnik, Amanda Blue, Justin Garrity, Dr. Byron Leak, Scot McCray, Pastor Vance Haywood, Dr. Peter Morris, Dr. Elizabeth Campbell, Peter Le, Lorena McDowell, Penny Washington, Shana Overdorf, Dr. Edwin Burkett, Peter Tannenbaum, Dean Mark Melton, Michael and Molly Painter, Amy Smith, Kim Crawford, Erin Yates, Brenda Gibson, Stephen Gruver, Sean Harrison, Dr. Dev Sangvai, Dr. Tara Lewis, Dr. Laura Gerald, Dr. Beat Steiner, Dr. Michael ZarZar, Julia Gamble, Tad Clodfelter, Anne Oshel, Dr. Michael Baca-Atlas, Daniel Lipparelli, Dr. Joel Lutterman, Deb Hueter, Ray Coppedge, Detective Wendy Clark, Maggie Kane, and the entire incredible staff at Place at the Table (dishing up daily doses of love, humanization, and delicious food—although honestly, I've never tried anything but the huevos rancheros, as it is too darn good). Thank you to Wake County's Robert Wood Johnson Scholars Thava Mahadevan, Dr. Derrick Hoover, WakeMed's very own Keturah Beckham, Dr. Jose Cabanas, and Jason Wittes who studied how to better collaborate across social sectors and better care for Wake County's familiar faces. And to all the amazing local independent doctors I have had a chance to learn from: Dr. Mary Forbes, Dr. Kenneth Holt, Dr. John Rubino, Dr. Prashant Patel, Dr. Stuart Levin, Dr. Conrad Flick, Rodger Israel, and the rest of the Key Physicians in Wake County.

Thank you to the incredible leadership at Oak City Cares, especially Kathy Johnson, Tosheria Brown, and Rick Miller-Haraway, who have built an incredible model of coordinating local efforts to help us manage the worsening issues around homelessness as a community.

Thank you also to all the leaders at North Carolina's Department of Human Health and Services—Cody Kinsley, Dr. Betsey Tilson, Mark Benton, and Dr. Mandy Cohen—who never stopped pushing to move our state in the right direction with Medicaid expansion and associated innovative care models. Your work built a culture of collaboration, support, and innovation.

To all the leadership at WakeMed who supported and helped to develop our work and innovation, including Becky Andrews (we never would have started this without your support), Dr. Bill Atkinson, Dr. West Lawson, Dr. Branson Page, Dr. Michael Watson, Dr. Tres Pittman, Linda Barrett, Sarah Hoffman, David Humes, Dr. Rasheeda Monroe, Dr. Micah Krempasky, Dr. John Holly, Dr. Theresa Amerson, Tina Morris-Anderson, Dr. Leslie McKinney, Dr. Carrie Dow Smith, Dr. Stephen Leinenweber, Dr. Chris DeRienzo, Dr. Matthew Nathan, Betsey McClain, Dr. Seth Brody, Christine Craig, Rick Shrum, Dee Darkes, Tom Klatt, Dr. Ami Rao-Zawadzki, Dr. Chuck Harr, Rick Carrico, and the rest of the hospital's staff and leaders. I am especially grateful to Donald Gintzig for his confident and determined leadership in prioritizing truly living up to our mission of serving the community and its most vulnerable residents.

I would also like to thank all our population health colleagues at both Duke University and University of North Carolina who have, over the years, prioritized collaboration to improve the outcomes in our shared communities, and Steve Lawler and the North Carolina Healthcare Association for creating a supportive environment for such innovative partnerships between health systems.

A very special thank you to Donna Avery, who has now been the architect of population health models spanning from "cradle to grave," from trauma-informed pediatric programs to our Center for Community Health, Innovation, and Equity serving the sickest in our community. She is always looking outward through the lens of innovation, with a focus on our most vulnerable residents. And to the Center staff: Dr. Annie Pugh, Shelby Shirley, Sheri Meinert, Penny Lockwood, Ty Whitehead, Beth Anne Downhower, Katrinka Mitchell, and Tricia Carr.

Thank you to Chelsea Bigelow, Chris Sikora, Sascha Godfrey, Mike Spadafora, Tommy Smith, and especially my editor, Jocelyn Carbonara, and project manager, Jenny Lisk, for helping me get this book over the finish line.

To my incredible family—wife, kids, parents, siblings, in-laws, nieces, and nephews—you are all truly the best; you make life awesome.

Finally, to my beautiful sister, Julie—you taught me not only how to celebrate life but, more importantly, *why* to celebrate life. You are a shining example of the love and goodness we all have the potential to bring into this world.

THE MEDICAL "GEEK-OUT" APPENDIX

APPENDIX 1
ACE SCREENING TOOL

aces aware

For Adults (Ages 18 and Older)

The **ACE Questionnaire for Adults** was adapted from the work of Kaiser Permanente and the Centers for Disease Control and Prevention (CDC). A version of the tool (Figure 5) has been compiled by the Office of the California Surgeon General and the Department of Health Care Services, in consultation with the ACEs Aware Clinical Advisory Subcommittee.

Figure 5. ACE Questionnaire for Adults — De-Identified

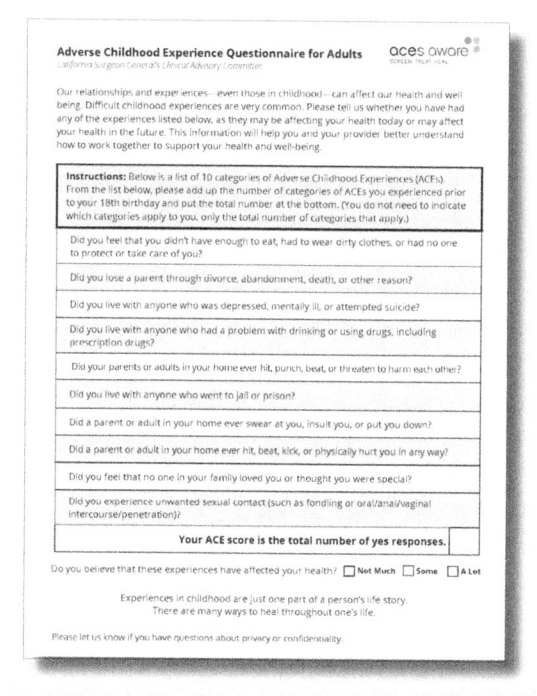

Adverse Childhood Experience Questionnaire for Adults
California Surgeon General's Clinical Advisory Committee

Our relationships and experiences—even those in childhood—can affect our health and well-being. Difficult childhood experiences are very common. Please tell us whether you have had any of the experiences listed below, as they may be affecting your health today or may affect your health in the future. This information will help you and your provider better understand how to work together to support your health and well-being.

Instructions: Below is a list of 10 categories of Adverse Childhood Experiences (ACEs). From the list below, please add up the number of categories of ACEs you experienced prior to your 18th birthday and put the total number at the bottom. (You do not need to indicate which categories apply to you, only the total number of categories that apply.)

Did you feel that you didn't have enough to eat, had to wear dirty clothes, or had no one to protect or take care of you?

Did you lose a parent through divorce, abandonment, death, or other reason?

Did you live with anyone who was depressed, mentally ill, or attempted suicide?

Did you live with anyone who had a problem with drinking or using drugs, including prescription drugs?

Did your parents or adults in your home ever hit, punch, beat, or threaten to harm each other?

Did you live with anyone who went to jail or prison?

Did a parent or adult in your home ever swear at you, insult you, or put you down?

Did a parent or adult in your home ever hit, beat, kick, or physically hurt you in any way?

Did you feel that no one in your family loved you or thought you were special?

Did you experience unwanted sexual contact (such as fondling or oral/anal/vaginal intercourse/penetration)?

Your ACE score is the total number of yes responses.

Do you believe that these experiences have affected your health? ☐ Not Much ☐ Some ☐ A Lot

Experiences in childhood are just one part of a person's life story.
There are many ways to heal throughout one's life.

Please let us know if you have questions about privacy or confidentiality.

APPENDIX 2
PATIENT INSIGHT, NOT LABELS

A few years ago, I had a visit from a patient who was barred from a local shelter, living in the woods, and suffering from addiction as he emotionally dealt with the recent overdose-related death of his partner of the past five years. He watched him die helplessly. His mental health screening in the clinic came back with "severe depression."

His simple response when I shared the results with him: "No shit, Sherlock."

In all patients, not just those suffering from homelessness, we encounter lives of loneliness, constant social dehumanization, and historic abuse. There's a danger of pathologizing and diagnosis-labeling what are ultimately inevitable symptoms resulting from lives of struggles and trauma. The temptation to define these symptoms simply as mental health diagnoses runs the risk of making patients feel sick and broken—of deflecting from the social realities of pain, isolation, and loneliness that are crushing them. It insinuates a pathologic, rather than a natural, response and can cycle back to reinforce feelings of brokenness.

The same is true about addiction. When does "a 15-times increased risk of substance abuse in a patient with five or more ACES" start being viewed as almost a natural consequence of experienced trauma as the body seeks relief? Or, as Dr. Daniel Sumrok, an addiction medicine specialist from the University of Tennessee describes it, "ritualized compulsive comfort-seeking." It's the neurologic equivalent of pulling your hand out of the fire, almost reflexively, to find relief and comfort from the intolerable pain of trauma. Those of us in healthcare need to address these root causes, the fire, and empower our patients with a more accurate perspective and insight—rather than just minimizing and mischaracterizing their realities by tossing out a diagnosis ... usually with an associated medication ... and often with a judgmental label.

Symptoms still absolutely need to be addressed clinically, but with care and thought. Medical providers and their teams must discuss with patients everything they are suffering through, their social issues, and their struggles. We need to help provide context for what they are feeling and how their bodies and minds are responding, so they can better understand and, hopefully and ideally, see strength in their resilience. We do this now routinely in our hotspotter clinic; it actually does not take long to provide at least a basic context and understanding, just as we would do with diabetes, hypertension, or any other medical condition.

People who suffer from trauma, mental health, addiction—any of them ... all of them—are some of the strongest people you'll ever meet. However, constant and relentless dehumanization, and their associated labels, can damage filters of self-perception to the point that it is almost impossible for a person to recognize their own beauty and strength.

If we can provide patients better insights into their symptoms, their history, and their illnesses—instead of just tossing out a 15-minute, hamster-wheel-produced diagnosis that pathologizes—then we can lay the foundation that empowers them to better address their mental health with, or if necessary without, the help of a broken health system that has historically ignored them. It's hard for a patient to address a condition they do not truly understand. It's our obligation as medical providers to make sure they do.

APPENDIX 3

CREATING MORE EFFICIENT AND ACCESSIBLE MENTAL HEALTH TOOLS FOR HISTORICALLY MARGINALIZED POPULATIONS

If we as medical providers don't have access to therapists and psychiatrists for our patients, we must adjust clinically to this reality and not get distracted by the temptations to just complain about it. Of course, on a larger scale, we need to be loud in advocating to fix a broken system, but we don't have the luxury of years, or generations, waiting for the changes we are advocating for. What can we do right now to help our patients expensively suffering and dying in front of us? Is there low-hanging fruit?

From a therapy perspective, is there another approach that can accomplish similar results—perhaps even at a lower cost? The history of medicine is riddled with examples where expensive, overly-complex, and long-accepted treatments, under the microscope of scientific rigor and examination, prove to be equivalent or even inferior to more simple and less complex alternatives. The business strategy that has been so successfully implemented throughout the years in medicine is to create this perceived complexity that justifies a costly, seemingly complex solution—ultimately, to create a dependency on these services that can then be expensively leveraged. It's a strategy for any business model: Create a dependency that you can then profit from, whether that be $7 caffe lattes, nicotine, video games, or healthcare. We, in medicine, keep our secrets close to the chest in an effort to create this perceived dependency. But the harms of keeping those secrets can be significant for those who cannot afford to hear them.

What if those secrets aren't as complex as we make them out to be? The fact is, they rarely are. And what if we, in medicine, share them—freely? While this is an unthinkable undermining of the foundational business strategy in fee-for-service models, it's the opposite in a "full-risk" value-based care model.

Some of the greatest innovations in medicine moving forward won't be mind-blowing technologic advances, allowing us to do the complex and dramatic even more complexly and dramatically. Lack of awesome technology is not one of the causes of medicine's current expensive inefficiencies. Rather, our greatest innovations will involve performing the simple, and therefore historically ignored, *better*.

On this note of simplicity, how do we empower patients to improve their own mental health through knowledge and awareness —through daily tools and routines they can use—so they don't feel that paying $200 per hour out of pocket to learn our secrets is their only option?

The current behavioral health shortage will remain for the near future, and it will disproportionately impact poor patients. It will result in disparities in mental health outcomes. How do we create an independence from, and alternative to, a system that has never been very successful in the first place? A strategy that can serve not only as a temporary solution but perhaps also provide insights into more permanent ones?

At the end of the pandemic, with behavioral issues spiking in our homeless populations and in populations of color,[1] our hotspotter team asked ourselves these very questions. As we worked with the uninsured and homeless, we realized that, except for a select few through intense advocacy, we were not going to get adequate access to behavioral health providers. We became interested in the growing literature around the benefits of telemedicine and virtual behavioral health apps that offered some hope in answering these questions[2]—at a very, very small fraction of the cost of traditional therapy. We were excited by the patient-empowerment and education focus on many of the apps—to empower their users with knowledge and education to help them better deal with stress and anxiety. We saw the utilization of such apps as a potentially viable and attractive option for broader population health initiatives at the community level, especially in Wake County, given our high uninsured rates at the time (pre-Medicaid expansion) that existed largely along racial lines. There were unique opportunities provided to us through partnerships to expand access to such apps in populations who may not otherwise have broad access to behavioral health resources.

Our team worked to gain access to thousands of subscriptions to a leading meditation app, not only in our clinic and hospital, but also out in the community with local medical, religious, and nonprofit organizations. Users were encouraged to engage with "daily mental health exercises"—for 8 to 10 minutes per day—preferably in the morning. We would ask them to avoid the temptation of hopping on their phones when they woke up to engage in often polarizing social media or news stories, and instead just focus on mindfulness, learning about recognizing when they are getting triggered, anxious, or depressed—the symptoms—and responding through meditation and related breathing techniques. These were daily neuroplasticity-based mental health exercises and lessons that could build up the "strength of the mind." We signed up more than 2,000 people, and the feedback was excellent.

I'm not saying it's *the* alternative to in-person therapy—I would argue, however, that it's much better than nothing. To work with patients to create more of an independence and autonomy from, not an expensive and manipulated dependency on, a system that historically failed them anyway.

Patient self-empowerment through knowledge has to become a foundational strategy in medicine moving forward—especially for historically marginalized populations.

APPENDIX 4

RIGHTING OUR HISTORIC WRONGS: THE POTENTIAL FOR MEDICAL EDUCATION TO HELP EVOLVE US CLOSER TO VOCATIONAL EFFICIENCY

There will likely always be massive waves in the break zones of medicine. And, in the foreseeable future, it looks like they will only get bigger. Even if we ride a few waves of success, there will always be other sets rolling in, constantly, that will keep us humble and fighting. They will keep pushing us under the water. Disparities. Inequities. HIV pandemic. COVID. Mental health crisis. The opioid epidemic. Housing affordability. Whatever is coming next.

As homeless numbers reach record highs nationally,[1] there are times when I finally feel like I am starting to drown a bit. I fear I'm getting pushed closer to what has always been my goal to avoid: burnout. It's why I have felt such an urgency in writing this book and expediting its publication. I already feel guilt for not doing it sooner. At Oak City Cares, open seats and space are hard to come by. Our shelters are out of beds. As in other cities across America, more and more tent communities are popping up locally in Raleigh. Our increased numbers are putting more pressure on our already strained safety nets. Growing populations equate to a growing number of poor outcomes. People are becoming fatigued. Fatigue facilitates the convenience of dehumanization.

We need more energy, innovation, and cognitive power in the break zone. We need more medical ingenuity. We need more people. This is the biggest challenge for us currently. How do we sustain our work while convincing others to jump in? How do we recruit into primary care ... much less public health ... much less homeless medicine?

It's not hard to rediscover purpose in the break zones of medicine; all you need to do is to look into the eyes of the patients who are found there, often clinging to you, desperate for help as they fight not to drown.

To be successful in the break zones, we must be comfortable in them. Teaching old dogs new tricks, especially when they are really stubborn, can be really hard. Possible, but really hard. Training future doctors and medical providers, so they are comfortable in the break zones of medicine as they enter their careers, may be the lower-hanging fruit. They are not blinded by our historic inefficiencies. There's the potential of idealism and new perspective to redirect trajectories through the possible, instead of simply sustaining them through the familiar yet inefficient.

Medicine is always evolving and learning. Science is always advancing.

WakeMed, led by the work of Dr. Rasheeda Monroe, has been participating in the University of North Carolina's Kenan Urban Scholars Program for years. Young student leaders participate in rotations after their first year of medical school, studying issues and complexities of urban medicine and developing a summer project. Dr. Monroe will not only share her work about ACEs, but also expose these students to the societal determinants of health and their impact. I have had the honor of mentoring in this program since 2020. It's motivating and inspirational to see future leaders of medicine with their idealism preserved and determined. It's fascinating to get their new, untainted perspectives through their research and projects on the inefficiencies in healthcare we have grown numb to.

They are the future leaders who will help determine where medicine goes from here. Will we finally bend the cost curve through improving our historic inefficiencies, or will simply expand these inefficiencies to push us further into unrecoverable debt, stealing resources and funding from other parts of society? Let their energy, idealism, and brilliance loose to help solve the chaos we created as their predecessors. Unleash their grit, and support it with purpose. But as we do so, we must create structures of support that can leverage purpose and passion. This includes reimbursement models that compensate providers for how they optimize health, not simply how they maximize procedures and services. We need to reward those who are committed to the vocation of medicine without demanding that they make personal and financial sacrifices in order to do so. We must empower them not to run away or become paralyzed in the break zone but rather to run into its waves, recklessly, and attack the chaos with their brilliance, humility, and determination. Have them lead the way and teach them to look around and appreciate the beauty in the entire process as they do so, from riding the occasional wave triumphantly to struggling with those that crash upon us unexpectedly. They can learn to celebrate the beauty in their colleagues who have chosen to be there battling with them, and the resilience in the patients they serve there.

This is how, as a profession, we as doctors will better live up to the vocational aspects and ideals of humanity inherent in the Hippocratic Oath that we all naively and obliviously swore to in our clean, starchy, costume-like, short white coats upon entering medicine.

NOTES

Introduction

1. "HUD Releases January 2023 Point-in-Time Count Report," *U.S. Department of Housing and Human Development*, December 15, 2023, https://www.hud.gov/press/press_releases_media_advisories/hud_no_23_278.
2. United States Interagency Council on Homelessness, "Homeless Courts: Recognizing Progress and Resolving Legal Issues That Often Accompany Homelessness," United States Interagency Council on Homelessness, July 9, 2020, https://www.usich.gov/news/homeless-courts-recognizing-progress-and-resolving-legal-issues-that-often-accompany-homelessness.
3. "Chronically Homeless," National Alliance to End Homelessness, December 18, 2023, https://endhomelessness.org/homelessness-in-america/who-experiences-homelessness/chronically-homeless.
4. "NHE Fact Sheet," CMS.gov, accessed July 15, 2024, https://www.cms.gov/data-research/statistics-trends-and-reports/national-health-expenditure-data/nhe-fact-sheet.

2. Mr. Spears

1. O'Connell, James J. MD. "Premature Mortality in Homeless Populations: A Review of the Literature." *National Health Care for the Homeless Council*, (2005): 13.

3. Vocation

1. Preeti Vankar, "US Health Expenditure as Percent of GDP from 1960 to 2022." Statista. February 16, 2024, https://www.statista.com/statistics/184968/us-health-expenditure-as-percent-of-gdp-since-1960
2. Julia La Roche, "Buffett: 'Medical Costs Are the Tapeworm of American Economic Competitiveness,'" Yahoo! Finance, accessed July 15, 2024, https://finance.yahoo.com/news/buffett-medical-costs-tapeworm-american-economic-competitiveness-220647855.html.
3. Robert Pear, "Clinton's Health Plan: The Overview; Congress Is Given the Clinton Plan for Health Care," *The New York Times*, October 28, 1993.
4. Bill Clinton, "Address of the President to the Joint Session of Congress," *U.S. Capitol* (speech, D.C., September 22, 1993).

4. The Costume

1. "Ancient Greek Medicine." U.S. National Library of Medicine. Accessed July 15, 2024. https://www.nlm.nih.gov/hmd/greek/greek_oath.html.

5. The Red Pill

1. Katrina Schwartz, "Four Pillars of a Meaningful Life That Could Be Part of Every Learning Community," KQED, December 10, 2018, https://www.kqed.org/mindshift/52620/four-pillars-of-a-meaningful-life-that-could-be-part-of-every-learning-community.

8. The Tapeworm

1. LeighAnne Olson, Robert S. Saunders, and Pierre L. Long, "The Healthcare Imperative: Lowering Costs and Improving Outcomes," *Institute of Medicine (US) Roundtable on Evidence-Based Medicine*, December 17, 2010, https://doi.org/10.17226/12750.
2. "Defining the Medical Home," Primary Care Collaborative, accessed March 13, 2024, https://thepcc.org/content/defining-medical-home
3. Jonathan Arend et al., "The Patient-centered Medical Home: History, Components, and Review of the Evidence," *Mount Sinai Journal of Medicine: A Journal of Translational and Personalized Medicine* 79, no. 4 (July 2012): 433–50, https://doi.org/10.1002/msj.21326.
4. Nisha Kurani and Cynthia Cox, "What Drives Health Spending in the U.S. Compared to Other Countries," Peterson-KFF Health System Tracker, July 20, 2021, https://www.healthsystemtracker.org/brief/what-drives-health-spending-in-the-u-s-compared-to-other-countries.
5. LeighAnne Olson, Robert S. Sanders, and Pierre L. Long, "The Healthcare Imperative: Lowering Costs and Improving Outcomes," *Institute of Medicine (US) Roundtable on Evidence-Based Medicine*, December 17, 2010, https://doi.org/10.17226/12750.
6. Monica Bharel et al., "Health Care Utilization Patterns of Homeless Individuals in Boston: Preparing for Medicaid Expansion under the Affordable Care Act," *American Journal of Public Health* 103, no. S2 (December 2013), https://doi.org/10.2105/ajph.2013.301421.
7. 2012 Published: May 01, "Health Care Costs: A Primer 2012 Report," KFF, July 25, 2014, https://www.kff.org/report-section/health-care-costs-a-primer-2012-report.
8. "Medicare Access and Chip Reauthorization Act (Macra), H.R. 2," Primary Care Collaborative, April 1, 2015, https://www.pcpcc.org/resource/medicare-access-and-chip-reauthorization-act-macra-hr-2.
9. James J. O'Connell, "Premature Mortality in Homeless Populations: A Review of the Literature," *National Health Care for the Homeless Council*, 2005.

12. Comfortably Broken

1. Carol K. Kane, "PRP: Recent Changes in Physician Practice Arrangements: Private Practice Dropped to Less Than 50 Percent of Physicians in 2020," Policy Research Perspectives, accessed July 16, 2024, https://www.ama-assn.org/system/files/2021-05/2020-prp-physician-practice-arrangements.pdf.

13. Hotspotting

1. Office of the Under Secretary of Defense, National Defense Budget Estimates for FY 2020 (2019).
2. "Fiscal Year 2010 Budget Summary—May 7, 2009," FY 2010 ED Budget Summary: Summary, accessed July 16, 2024, https://www2.ed.gov/about/overview/budget/budget10/summary/edlite-section1.html.
3. Steven A. Schroeder, "We Can Do Better—Improving the Health of the American People," *New England Journal of Medicine* 357, no. 12 (September 20, 2007): 1221–28, https://doi.org/10.1056/nejmsa073350.
4. Atul Gawande, "Finding Medicine's Hot Spots," *The New Yorker*, January 17, 2011, https://www.newyorker.com/magazine/2011/01/24/the-hot-spotters.

14. Bloodletting and Dirty Hands

1. PBS News Hour, "Bloodletting and Blisters: Solving the Medical Mystery of George Washington's Death," PBS, December 16, 2014, https://www.pbs.org/newshour/show/bloodletting-blisters-solving-medical-mystery-george-washingtons-death.
2. "The Death of George Washington," George Washington's Mount Vernon, accessed July 15, 2024, https://www.mountvernon.org/library/digitalhistory/digital-encyclopedia/article/the-death-of-george-washington.
3. Larry Getlen, "The Inept Doctor Who Killed President Garfield," *New York Post*, September 23, 2016, https://nypost.com/2016/09/22/the-inept-doctor-who-killed-president-garfield.
4. Zoë Slote Morris, Steven Wooding, and Jonathan Grant, "The Answer Is 17 Years, What Is the Question: Understanding Time Lags in Translational Research," *Journal of the Royal Society of Medicine* 104, no. 12 (December 2011): 510–20, https://doi.org/10.1258/jrsm.2011.110180.
5. Jonathan P. Weiner et al., "In-Person and Telehealth Ambulatory Contacts and Costs in a Large US Insured Cohort before and during the COVID-19 Pandemic," *JAMA Network Open* 4, no. 3 (March 23, 2021), https://doi.org/10.1001/jamanetworkopen.2021.2618.

16. Aha

1. Daniel Flaming and Halil Toros, "Silicon Valley Triage Tool," Economic roundtable, February 17, 2016, https://economicrt.org/publication/silicon-valley-triage-tool.
2. rep., *Wake County Population Health Task Force* (Wake County, NC, 2018).
3. "About Adverse Childhood Experiences," Centers for Disease Control and Prevention, May 16, 2024, https://www.cdc.gov/aces/about/index.html.
4. Working paper, *Early Experiences Can Alter Gene Expression and Affect Long-Term Development*, 2010.
5. "Understanding the Impact of Adverse Childhood Experiences (ACEs)," Center

for Youth Wellness, June 26, 2024, https://centerforyouthwellness.org/wp-content/themes/cyw/build/img/building-a-movement/hidden-crisis.pdf.
6. Katherine A. Koh and Ann Elizabeth Montgomery, "Adverse Childhood Experiences and Homelessness: Advances and Aspirations," *The Lancet Public Health* 6, no. 11 (November 2021), https://doi.org/10.1016/s2468-2667(21)00210-3.
7. Travis P. Baggett et al., "Mortality among Homeless Adults in Boston," *JAMA Internal Medicine* 173, no. 3 (February 11, 2013): 189, https://doi.org/10.1001/jamainternmed.2013.1604.
8. Vincent J. Felitti et al., "Relationship of Childhood Abuse and Household Dysfunction to Many of the Leading Causes of Death in Adults," *American Journal of Preventive Medicine* 14, no. 4 (May 1998): 245–58, https://doi.org/10.1016/s0749-3797(98)00017-8.
9. "What Are Adverse Childhood Experiences (Aces)?," WAVE Trust, accessed July 15, 2024, https://www.wavetrust.org/adverse-childhood-experiences.

19. Reflexive Dehumanization

1. William St. Clair, *The Grand Slave Emporium: Cape Coast Castle and the British Slave Trade* (London: Profile Books, 2006).
2. The German Churches and the Nazi State," United States Holocaust Memorial Museum, accessed July 17, 2024, https://encyclopedia.ushmm.org/content/en/article/the-german-churches-and-the-nazi-state.
3. Lasana T. Harris and Susan T. Fiske, "Dehumanized Perception," *Zeitschrift Für Psychologie* 219, no. 3 (January 2011): 175–81, https://doi.org/10.1027/2151-2604/a000065.
4. "Brain's Failure to Appreciate Others May Permit Human Atrocities," ScienceDaily, December 15, 2011, https://www.sciencedaily.com/releases/2011/12/111214162103.htm.

20. Social Hierarchy

1. Jessica E. Koski, Hongling Xie, and Ingrid R. Olson, "Understanding Social Hierarchies: The Neural and Psychological Foundations of Status Perception," *Social Neuroscience* 10, no. 5 (February 20, 2015): 527–50, https://doi.org/10.1080/17470919.2015.1013223.
2. Paul K. Piff et al., "Higher Social Class Predicts Increased Unethical Behavior," *Proceedings of the National Academy of Sciences* 109, no. 11 (February 27, 2012): 4086–91, https://doi.org/10.1073/pnas.1118373109.
3. Robert B. Lount and Nathan C. Pettit, "The Social Context of Trust: The Role of Status," *Organizational Behavior and Human Decision Processes* 117, no. 1 (January 2012): 15–23, https://doi.org/10.1016/j.obhdp.2011.07.005.
4. Andrew Huberman, "Science of Social Bonding in Family, Friendship & Romantic Love," Huberman Lab, December 19, 2021, https://www.hubermanlab.com/episode/science-of-social-bonding-in-family-friendship-and-romantic-love.
5. Lotte Thomsen, "The Developmental Origins of Social Hierarchy: How Infants and Young Children Mentally Represent and Respond to Power and Status,"

Current Opinion in Psychology 33 (June 2020): 201–8, https://doi.org/10.1016/j.copsyc.2019.07.044.
6. Franchesca Ramirez et al., "Active Avoidance Requires a Serial Basal Amygdala to Nucleus Accumbens Shell Circuit," *The Journal of Neuroscience* 35, no. 8 (February 25, 2015): 3470–77, https://doi.org/10.1523/jneurosci.1331-14.2015.

21. Loneliness

1. Robert Waldinger, "What Makes a Good Life? Lessons from the Longest Study on Happiness," *TedxBeaconStreet*, (lecture, n.d.), https://www.ted.com/talks/robert_waldinger_what_makes_a_good_life_lessons_from_the_longest_study_on_happiness?subtitle=en&trigger=30s.
2. Office of the Assistant Secretary for Health (OASH), "New Surgeon General Advisory Raises Alarm about the Devastating Impact of the Epidemic of Loneliness and Isolation in the United States," HHS.gov, May 3, 2023, https://www.hhs.gov/about/news/2023/05/03/new-surgeon-general-advisory-raises-alarm-about-devastating-impact-epidemic-loneliness-isolation-united-states.html.
3. Ryo Naito et al., "Social Isolation as a Risk Factor for All-Cause Mortality: Systematic Review and Meta-Analysis of Cohort Studies," *PLOS ONE* 18, no. 1 (January 12, 2023), https://doi.org/10.1371/journal.pone.0280308.

22. Twenty-Seven Pounds of Chains

1. Angela Browne and Shari S. Bassuk, "Intimate Violence in the Lives of Homeless and Poor Housed Women: Prevalence and Patterns in an Ethnically Diverse Sample.," *American Journal of Orthopsychiatry* 67, no. 2 (1997): 261–78, https://doi.org/10.1037/h0080230.
2. Suzanne L. Wenzel, Barbara D. Leake, and Lillian Gelberg, "Health of Homeless Women with Recent Experience of Rape," *Journal of General Internal Medicine* 15, no. 4 (April 2000): 265–68, https://doi.org/10.1111/j.1525-1497.2000.04269.x.
3. Richard J. Estes and Neil Alan Weiner, "Commercial Sexual Exploitation of Children in the United States, 1997-2000," *ICPSR Data Holdings*, March 27, 2003, https://doi.org/10.3886/icpsr03366.v1.
4. Housing, Homelessness, and Sexual Violence Statistics accessed July 17, 2024, https://www.nsvrc.org/sites/default/files/NSAC11_Handouts/NSAC11_Handout_With_Statistics.pdf.
5. Lauren Abern et al., "Sexual Assault and Homelessness in the Transgender Population: Are We Doing Enough? [A309]," *Obstetrics & Gynecology* 139, no. 1 (May 2022), https://doi.org/10.1097/01.aog.0000825556.22843.02.
6. Rebecca L. Gibson and Timothy S. Hartshorne, "Childhood Sexual Abuse and Adult Loneliness and Network Orientation," *Child Abuse & Neglect* 20, no. 11 (November 1996): 1087–93, https://doi.org/10.1016/0145-2134(96)00097-x.
7. Amy M. Young, Carol Boyd, and Amy Hubbell, "Social Isolation & Sexual Abuse among Women Who Smoke Crack," *Journal of Psychosocial Nursing and Mental Health Services* 39, no. 7 (July 2001): 12–20, https://doi.org/10.3928/0279-3695-20010701-10.

23. The Beam

1. William H. Shrank, Teresa L. Rogstad, and Natasha Parekh, "Waste in the US Health Care System," *JAMA* 322, no. 15 (October 15, 2019): 1501, https://doi.org/10.1001/jama.2019.13978.
2. Martin A Makary and Michael Daniel, "Medical Error—the Third Leading Cause of Death in the US," *BMJ*, May 3, 2016, i2139, https://doi.org/10.1136/bmj.i2139.
3. Jon B. Christianson et al., "Physician Communication with Patients: Research Findings and Challenge," *Health Policy and Management, University of Minnesota* 29, no. 4 (2012).
4. Sade Udoetuk, Deepa Dongarwar, and Hamisu M. Salihu, "Racial and Gender Disparities in Diagnosis of Malingering in Clinical Settings," *Journal of Racial and Ethnic Health Disparities* 7, no. 6 (March 9, 2020): 1117–23, https://doi.org/10.1007/s40615-020-00734-6.

24. The Four Rs

1. Jaclyn N. Portelli Tremont, Brian Klausner, and Pascal Osita Udekwu, "Embracing a Trauma-Informed Approach to Patient Care—in with the New," *JAMA Surgery* 156, no. 12 (December 1, 2021): 1083, https://doi.org/10.1001/jamasurg.2021.4284.
2. Office of Policy, Planning, and Innovation, SAMHSA's Concept of Trauma and Guidance for a Trauma-Informed Approach (2014).

25. Listen

1. Lasana T. Harris and Susan T. Fiske, "Dehumanized Perception," *Zeitschrift Für Psychologie* 219, no. 3 (January 2011): 175–81, https://doi.org/10.1027/2151-2604/a000065.
2. Katy Johnston and Hannah Westwater, "Why Is Empathy for Homeless People Lacking? Science," *Street Roots*, July 30, 2019, https://www.streetroots.org/news/2019/07/26/why-empathy-homeless-people-lacking-science.
3. Katy Johnston and Hannah Westwater, "This Is Your Brain on Homelessness," Big Issue, January 25, 2019, https://www.bigissue.com/news/housing/this-is-your-brain-on-homelessness.
4. Katy Johnston and Hannah Westwater, "This Is Your Brain on Homelessness," *Big Issue*, January 25, 2019, https://www.bigissue.com/news/housing/this-is-your-brain-on-homelessness.
5. Naykky Singh Ospina et al., "Eliciting the Patient's Agenda- Secondary Analysis of Recorded Clinical Encounters," *Journal of General Internal Medicine* 34, no. 1 (July 2, 2018): 36–40, https://doi.org/10.1007/s11606-018-4540-5.

26. Feeding the Fire While Fighting the Flame

1. Gary Claxton et al., "Health Benefits in 2021: Employer Programs Evolving in Response to the COVID-19 Pandemic," *Health Affairs* 40, no. 12 (December 1, 2021): 1961–71, https://doi.org/10.1377/hlthaff.2021.01503.
2. Noam N. Levey, "Few Places Have More Medical Debt than Dallas-Fort Worth, but Hospitals There Are Thriving," KFF Health News, September 30, 2022, https://khn.org/news/article/medical-debt-hospitals-dallas-fort-worth.
3. Bronwen Lichtenstein and Joe Weber, "Losing Ground: Racial Disparities in Medical Debt and Home Foreclosure in the Deep South. Fam Community Health," *Family & Community Health* 39, no. 3 (July 2016): 178–87, https://doi.org/10.1097/fch.0000000000000108.

27. Disparities

1. "Story Map Series," unc.maps.arcgis.com, accessed July 15, 2024, https://unc.maps.arcgis.com/apps/MapSeries/index.html.
2. "North Carolina: All Race & Ethnicity Data," The COVID Tracking Project, accessed July 15, 2024, https://covidtracking.com/data/state/north-carolina/race-ethnicity.
3. "New Maps Show Differences in Life Expectancy." North Carolina Health News, August 5, 2015. https://www.northcarolinahealthnews.org/2015/08/05/new-maps-show-differences-in-life-expectancy.
4. "Homelessness and Racial Disparities," National Alliance to End Homelessness, December 18, 2023, https://endhomelessness.org/homelessness-in-america/what-causes-homelessness/inequality.
5. Point in Time Data—2021—Wake Continuum of Care—NC 507, accessed July 16, 2024, https://wakecoc.org/data/pit-2021.
6. "2022 APM Measurement Infographic," Health Care Payment Learning & Action Network - Quality Care, Improved Health, and Lower Costs, July 7, 2023, https://hcp-lan.org/apm-measurement-effort/2022-apm/2022-infographic/.
7. "Innovation Center Strategy Refresh," Centers for Medicare and Medicaid Services, accessed July 16, 2024, https://www.cms.gov/priorities/innovation/strategic-direction-whitepaper.
8. Katarzyna Bryc et al., "The Genetic Ancestry of African Americans, Latinos, and European Americans across the United States," American Journal of Human Genetics, January 8, 2015, https://www.ncbi.nlm.nih.gov/pmc/articles/PMC4289685.
9. Bhatt, Jay, Wendy Gerhardt, Andy Davis FSA, MAAA, Neal Batra, Dr. Asif Dhar, and Brian Rush, "US Health Care Can't Afford Health Inequities," *Deloitte Insights*, June 22, 2022. https://www2.deloitte.com/us/en/insights/industry/health-care/economic-cost-of-health-disparities.html.

28. Mental Health

1. Daniel Goleman, "Sad Legacy of Abuse: The Search for Remedies," The New York Times, January 24, 1989, https://www.nytimes.com/1989/01/24/science/sad-legacy-of-abuse-the-search-for-remedies.html.
2. M. Glasser et al., "Cycle of Child Sexual Abuse: Links between Being a Victim and Becoming a Perpetrator," *British Journal of Psychiatry* 179, no. 6 (December 2001): 482–94, https://doi.org/10.1192/bjp.179.6.482.
3. rep., *The Silent Shortage: A White Paper Examining Supply, Demand and Recruitment Trends in Psychiatry*, White Paper Series (Merritt Hawkins, 2018).
4. Tara F. Bishop et al., "Acceptance of Insurance by Psychiatrists and the Implications for Access to Mental Health Care," *JAMA Psychiatry* 71, no. 2 (February 1, 2014): 176, https://doi.org/10.1001/jamapsychiatry.2013.2862.
5. "Behavioral Health Patients Spur 57% of Commercial Healthcare Spending," *Modern Healthcare*, accessed July 16, 2024, https://www.modernhealthcare.com/patient-care/behavioral-health-patients-spur-57-commercial-healthcare-spending.
6. Eric Lopez et al., "How Much More Than Medicare Do Private Insurers Pay? A Review of the Literature," *KFF*, April 15, 2020.
7. Tara F. Bishop et al., "Acceptance of Insurance by Psychiatrists and the Implications for Access to Mental Health Care," *JAMA Psychiatry* 71, no. 2 (February 1, 2014): 176, https://doi.org/10.1001/jamapsychiatry.2013.2862.
8. Thomas G. McGuire and Jeanne Miranda, "New Evidence Regarding Racial and Ethnic Disparities in Mental Health: Policy Implications," *Health Affairs* 27, no. 2 (March 2008): 393–403, https://doi.org/10.1377/hlthaff.27.2.393.
9. Rabah Kamal and Gary Claxton, "Exploring Mental and Behavioral Health and Substance Abuse," Peterson-KFF Health System Tracker, May 5, 2016, https://www.healthsystemtracker.org/brief/exploring-mental-and-behavioral-health-and-substance-abuse.
10. Stoddard Davenport, T.J. Gray, and Steve Melek, "How Do Individuals with Behavioral Health Conditions Contribute to Physical and Total Healthcare Spending?," *Milliman Research Report*, August 13, 2020.
11. Stephen P Melek et al., "Whole-Person Health Care: Integrating Mental and Behavioral Health Into Primary Care," *The American Journal of Managed Care* (lecture, October 16, 2020).

29. Justice System

1. U.S. Department of Justice and Caroline Wolf Harlow, Education and Correctional Populations (2003).
2. Executive Office of the President of the United States, The State of Homelessness in America (2019).
3. Lucius Couloute, "Nowhere to Go: Homelessness among Formerly Incarcerated People," Prison Policy Initiative, August 2018, https://www.prisonpolicy.org/reports/housing.html.
4. Doris J. James, "Profile of Jail Inmates, 2002—Bureau of Justice Statistics," US Department of Justice, 2002, https://bjs.ojp.gov/content/pub/pdf/pji02.pdf.

5. Janey Rountree, Austen Lyke, and Nathan Hess, "Health Conditions among Unsheltered Adults in the U.S.," California Policy Lab, October 6, 2019, https://capolicylab.org/health-conditions-among-unsheltered-adults-in-the-u-s.
6. M M Loomans, J H M Tulen, and H J C. van Marle, "The Neurobiology of Antisocial Behaviour," *Tijdschr Psychiatr*, 2010.
7. Maureen Buell, Stephanie S. Covington, and Nena Messina, "The Association between ACEs and Criminal Justice Involvement, Part 1," *Becoming Trauma Informed: An Essential Element for Justice Settings* (lecture, July 16, 2024).
8. United States Interagency Council on Homelessness, "Homeless Courts: Recognizing Progress and Resolving Legal Issues That Often Accompany Homelessness," United States Interagency Council on Homelessness, July 9, 2020, https://www.usich.gov/news/homeless-courts-recognizing-progress-and-resolving-legal-issues-that-often-accompany-homelessness.
9. Helen Fair and Roy Walmsley, rep., *World Prison Population List (Thirteenth Edition)* (World Prison Brief, n.d.).
10. United States Interagency Council on Homelessness, "Homeless Courts: Recognizing Progress and Resolving Legal Issues That Often Accompany Homelessness," United States Interagency Council on Homelessness, July 9, 2020, https://www.usich.gov/news/homeless-courts-recognizing-progress-and-resolving-legal-issues-that-often-accompany-homelessness.
11. Holley Davis, "Meeting Health Needs at Reentry: North Carolina's Fit Program," Policy Research Associates, October 14, 2021, https://www.prainc.com/gains-north-carolina-fit-program.
12. Helen Fair and Roy Walmsley, rep., *World Prison Population List (Thirteenth Edition)* (World Prison Brief, n.d.).

30. One Nation

1. Mary E. Larimer et al., "Health Care and Public Service Use and Costs before and after Provision of Housing for Chronically Homeless Persons with Severe Alcohol Problems," *JAMA* 301, no. 13 (April 1, 2009): 1349, https://doi.org/10.1001/jama.2009.414.

31. Under God

1. "How Religious Are Americans?" Gallup, March 29, 2024, https://news.gallup.com/poll/358364/religious-americans.aspx.
2. Patricia L. Lockwood, "The Anatomy of Empathy: Vicarious Experience and Disorders of Social Cognition," *Behavioural Brain Research* 311 (September 2016): 255–66, https://doi.org/10.1016/j.bbr.2016.05.048.
3. Alexandra Touroutoglou et al., "The Tenacious Brain: How the Anterior Mid-Cingulate Contributes to Achieving Goals," *Cortex* 123 (February 2020): 12–29, https://doi.org/10.1016/j.cortex.2019.09.011.
4. Hui BPH; Ng JCK; Berzaghi E; Cunningham-Amos LA; Kogan A., "Rewards of Kindness? A Meta-Analysis of the Link between Prosociality and Well-Being," Psychological bulletin, accessed July 15, 2024, https://pubmed.ncbi.nlm.nih.gov/32881540.

5. Thomas Oppong, "Aristotle's Principles for a Good Life," *Medium*, September 21, 2022, https://medium.com/personal-growth/aristotles-principles-for-a-good-life-9f474a5f02bc.

33. In the End

1. Linda K. George et al., "Spirituality and Health: What We Know, What We Need to Know," *Journal of Social and Clinical Psychology* 19, no. 1 (March 2000): 102–16, https://doi.org/10.1521/jscp.2000.19.1.102.

Appendix 3

1. Alyssa Flowers and William Wan, "Depression and Anxiety Spiked among Black Americans after George Floyd's Death," *The Washington Post*, June 12, 2020.
2. Jake Linardon et al., "The Efficacy of Mindfulness Apps on Symptoms of Depression and Anxiety: An Updated Meta-Analysis of Randomized Controlled Trials," *Clinical Psychology Review* 107 (February 2024): 102370, https://doi.org/10.1016/j.cpr.2023.102370.

Appendix 4

1. "State of Homelessness: 2023 Edition," National Alliance to End Homelessness, January 6, 2024, https://endhomelessness.org/homelessness-in-america/homelessness-statistics/state-of-homelessness.

BIBLIOGRAPHY

"2022 APM Measurement Infographic." Health Care Payment Learning & Action Network—Quality Care, Improved Health, and Lower Costs, July 7, 2023. https://hcp-lan.org/apm-measurement-effort/2022-apm/2022-infographic/.

Abern, Lauren, Chance Krempasky, Daniela Diego, and Karla Maguire. "Sexual Assault and Homelessness in the Transgender Population: Are We Doing Enough? [A309]." *Obstetrics & Gynecology* 139, no. 1 (May 2022). https://doi.org/10.1097/01.aog.0000825556.22843.02.

"About Adverse Childhood Experiences." Centers for Disease Control and Prevention, May 16, 2024. https://www.cdc.gov/aces/about/index.html.

"Ancient Greek Medicine." U.S. National Library of Medicine. Accessed July 15, 2024. https://www.nlm.nih.gov/hmd/greek/greek_oath.html.

Arend, Jonathan, Jenny Tsang-Quinn, Claudia Levine, and David Thomas. "The Patient-centered Medical Home: History, Components, and Review of the Evidence." *Mount Sinai Journal of Medicine: A Journal of Translational and Personalized Medicine* 79, no. 4 (July 2012): 433–50. https://doi.org/10.1002/msj.21326.

Baggett, Travis P., Stephen W. Hwang, James J. O'Connell, Bianca C. Porneala, Erin J. Stringfellow, E. John Orav, Daniel E. Singer, and Nancy A. Rigotti. "Mortality among Homeless Adults in Boston." *JAMA Internal Medicine* 173, no. 3 (February 11, 2013): 189. https://doi.org/10.1001/jamainternmed.2013.1604.

"Behavioral Health Patients Spur 57% of Commercial Healthcare Spending." *Modern Healthcare*. Accessed July 16, 2024. https://www.modernhealthcare.com/patient-care/behavioral-health-patients-spur-57-commercial-healthcare-spending.

Bharel, Monica, Wen-Chieh Lin, Jianying Zhang, Elizabeth O'Connell, Robert Taube, and Robin E. Clark. "Health Care Utilization Patterns of Homeless Individuals in Boston: Preparing for Medicaid Expansion under the Affordable Care Act." *American Journal of Public Health* 103, no. S2 (December 2013). https://doi.org/10.2105/ajph.2013.301421.

Bhatt, Jay, Wendy Gerhardt, Andy Davis FSA, MAAA, Neal Batra, Dr. Asif Dhar, and Brian Rush. "U.S. Health Care Can't Afford Health Inequities." *Deloite Insights*, June 22, 2022. https://www2.deloitte.com/us/en/insights/industry/health-care/economic-cost-of-health-disparities.html.

Bishop, Tara F., Matthew J. Press, Salomeh Keyhani, and Harold Alan Pincus. "Acceptance of Insurance by Psychiatrists and the Implications for Access to Mental Health Care." *JAMA Psychiatry* 71, no. 2 (February 1, 2014): 176. https://doi.org/10.1001/jamapsychiatry.2013.2862.

Boyles, Greg. 2011. *Tattoos on the Heart: The Power of Boundless Compassion*. Washington, DC: Free Press.

"Brain's Failure to Appreciate Others May Permit Human Atrocities." ScienceDaily,

December 15, 2011. https://www.sciencedaily.com/releases/2011/12/111214162103.htm.

Browne, Angela, and Shari S. Bassuk. "Intimate Violence in the Lives of Homeless and Poor Housed Women: Prevalence and Patterns in an Ethnically Diverse Sample." *American Journal of Orthopsychiatry* 67, no. 2 (1997): 261–78. https://doi.org/10.1037/h0080230.

Bryc, Katarzyna, Eric Y. Durand, J. Michael Macpherson, David Reich, and Joanna L. Mountain. "The Genetic Ancestry of African Americans, Latinos, and European Americans across the United States." *American Journal of Human Genetics*, January 8, 2015. https://www.ncbi.nlm.nih.gov/pmc/articles/PMC4289685.

Buell, Maureen, Stephanie S Covington, and Nena Messina. "The Association between ACEs and Criminal Justice Involvement, Part 1." *Becoming Trauma Informed: An Essential Element for Justice Settings*. Lecture presented at the National Institute of Corrections (NIC), July 16, 2024.

Christianson, Jon B., Wayne Jonas, Michael Finch, and Louise H Warrick. "Physician Communication with Patients: Research Findings and Challenge." *Health Policy and Management, University of Minnesota* 29, no. 4 (2012).

"Chronically Homeless." National Alliance to End Homelessness, December 18, 2023. https://endhomelessness.org/homelessness-in-america/who-experiences-homelessness/chronically-homeless.

Claxton, Gary, Matthew Rae, Anthony Damico, Gregory Young, Nisha Kurani, and Heidi Whitmore. "Health Benefits in 2021: Employer Programs Evolving in Response to the COVID-19 Pandemic." *Health Affairs* 40, no. 12 (December 1, 2021): 1961–71. https://doi.org/10.1377/hlthaff.2021.01503.

Clinton, Bill. "Address of the President to the Joint Session of Congress." *U.S. Capitol*. Speech presented at the Speech by President Address to Joint Session of Congress as Delivered, September 22, 1993.

Couloute, Lucius. "Nowhere to Go: Homelessness among Formerly Incarcerated People." Prison Policy Initiative, August 2018. https://www.prisonpolicy.org/reports/housing.html.

Davenport, Stoddard, T.J. Gray, and Steve Melek. "How Do Individuals with Behavioral Health Conditions Contribute to Physical and Total Healthcare Spending?" *Milliman Research Report*, August 13, 2020.

Davis, Holley. "Meeting Health Needs at Reentry: North Carolina's Fit Program." Policy Research Associates, October 14, 2021. https://www.prainc.com/gains-north-carolina-fit-program.

"The Death of George Washington." George Washington's Mount Vernon. Accessed July 15, 2024. https://www.mountvernon.org/library/digitalhistory/digital-encyclopedia/article/the-death-of-george-washington.

"Defining the Medical Home." Primary Care Collaborative. Accessed July 15, 2024. https://thepcc.org/content/defining-medical-home.

Estes, Richard J., and Neil Alan Weiner. "Commercial Sexual Exploitation of Children in the United States, 1997-2000." *ICPSR Data Holdings*, March 27, 2003. https://doi.org/10.3886/icpsr03366.v1.

Executive Office of the President of the United States, "The State of Homelessness in America" (2019).

Fair, Helen, and Roy Walmsley. Rep. *World Prison Population List (Thirteenth Edition)*. World Prison Brief, n.d.

Felitti, Vincent J., Robert F. Anda, Dale Nordenberg, David F. Williamson, Alison M. Spitz, Valerie Edwards, Mary P. Koss, and James S. Marks. "Relationship of Childhood Abuse and Household Dysfunction to Many of the Leading Causes of Death in Adults." *American Journal of Preventive Medicine* 14, no. 4 (May 1998): 245–58. https://doi.org/10.1016/s0749-3797(98)00017-8.

"Fiscal Year 2010 Budget Summary—May 7, 2009." FY 2010 ED Budget Summary: Summary. Accessed July 16, 2024. https://www2.ed.gov/about/overview/budget/budget10/summary/edlite-section1.html.

Flaming, Daniel, and Halil Toros. "Silicon Valley Triage Tool." Economic Roundtable, February 17, 2016. https://economicrt.org/publication/silicon-valley-triage-tool.

Flowers, Alyssa, and William Wan. "Depression and Anxiety Spiked among Black Americans after George Floyd's Death." *The Washington Post*, June 12, 2020.

Gawande, Atul. "Finding Medicine's Hot Spots." The New Yorker, January 17, 2011. https://www.newyorker.com/magazine/2011/01/24/the-hot-spotters.

George, Linda K., David B. Larson, Harold G. Koenig, and Michael E. McCullough. "Spirituality and Health: What We Know, What We Need to Know." *Journal of Social and Clinical Psychology* 19, no. 1 (March 2000): 102–16. https://doi.org/10.1521/jscp.2000.19.1.102.

"The German Churches and the Nazi State." United States Holocaust Memorial Museum. Accessed July 17, 2024. https://encyclopedia.ushmm.org/content/en/article/the-german-churches-and-the-nazi-state.

Getlen, Larry. "The Inept Doctor Who Killed President Garfield." *New York Post*, September 23, 2016. https://nypost.com/2016/09/22/the-inept-doctor-who-killed-president-garfield.

Gibson, Rebecca L., and Timothy S. Hartshorne. "Childhood Sexual Abuse and Adult Loneliness and Network Orientation." *Child Abuse & Neglect* 20, no. 11 (November 1996): 1087–93. https://doi.org/10.1016/0145-2134(96)00097-x.

Glasser, M., I. Kolvin, D. Campbell, A. Glasser, I. Leitch, and S. Farrelly. "Cycle of Child Sexual Abuse: Links between Being a Victim and Becoming a Perpetrator." *British Journal of Psychiatry* 179, no. 6 (December 2001): 482–94. https://doi.org/10.1192/bjp.179.6.482.

Goleman, Daniel. "Sad Legacy of Abuse: The Search for Remedies." *The New York Times*, January 24, 1989. https://www.nytimes.com/1989/01/24/science/sad-legacy-of-abuse-the-search-for-remedies.html.

Harris, Lasana T., and Susan T. Fiske. "Dehumanized Perception." *Zeitschrift für Psychologie* 219, no. 3 (January 2011): 175–81. https://doi.org/10.1027/2151-2604/a000065.

"Homelessness and Racial Disparities." National Alliance to End Homelessness, December 18, 2023. https://endhomelessness.org/homelessness-in-america/what-causes-homelessness/inequality.

Hour, PBS News. "Bloodletting and Blisters: Solving the Medical Mystery of George Washington's Death." PBS, December 16, 2014. https://www.pbs.org/newshour/show/bloodletting-blisters-solving-medical-mystery-george-washing tons-death.

Housing, Homelessness, and Sexual Violence Statistics. Accessed July 17, 2024. https://www.nsvrc.org/sites/default/files/NSAC11_Handouts/NSAC11_Handout_With_Statistics.pdf.

"How Religious Are Americans?" Gallup, March 29, 2024. https://news.gallup.com/poll/358364/religious-americans.aspx.

Huberman, Andrew. "David Goggins: How to Build Immense Inner Strength." YouTube, January 1, 2024. https://www.youtube.com/watch?v=nDLb8_wgX50.

Huberman, Andrew. "Science of Social Bonding in Family, Friendship & Romantic Love." Huberman Lab, December 19, 2021. https://www.hubermanlab.com/episode/science-of-social-bonding-in-family-friendship-and-romantic-love.

"HUD Releases January 2023 Point-in-Time Count Report." *U.S. Department of Housing and Human Development*, December 15, 2023. https://www.hud.gov/press/press_releases_media_advisories/hud_no_23_278.

Hui BPH; Ng JCK; Berzaghi E; Cunningham-Amos LA; Kogan A; "Rewards of Kindness? A Meta-Analysis of the Link between Prosociality and Well-Being." Psychological bulletin. Accessed July 15, 2024. https://pubmed.ncbi.nlm.nih.gov/32881540.

"Innovation Center Strategy Refresh." Centers for Medicare and Medicaid Services. Accessed July 16, 2024. https://www.cms.gov/priorities/innovation/strategic-direction-whitepaper.

James, Doris J. "Profile of Jail Inmates, 2002—Bureau of Justice Statistics." US Department of Justice, 2002. https://bjs.ojp.gov/content/pub/pdf/pji02.pdf.

Johnston, Katy, and Hannah Westwater. "This Is Your Brain on Homelessness." Big Issue, January 25, 2019. https://www.bigissue.com/news/housing/this-is-your-brain-on-homelessness.

Johnston, Katy, and Hannah Westwater. "Why Is Empathy for Homeless People Lacking? Science." *Street Roots*, July 30, 2019. https://www.streetroots.org/news/2019/07/26/why-empathy-homeless-people-lacking-science.

Kamal, Rabah, and Gary Claxton. "Exploring Mental and Behavioral Health and Substance Abuse." Peterson-KFF Health System Tracker, May 5, 2016. https://www.healthsystemtracker.org/brief/exploring-mental-and-behavioral-health-and-substance-abuse.

Kidder, Tracey. *Rough Sleepers: Dr. Jim O'Connell's Urgent Mission to Bring Healing to Homeless People*. New York: Penguin Random House, 2023.

Kane, Carol K. "PRP: Recent Changes in Physician Practice Arrangements: Private Practice Dropped to Less Than 50 Percent of Physicians in 2020." *Policy Research Perspectives*. Accessed July 16, 2024. https://www.ama-assn.org/system/files/2021-05/2020-prp-physician-practice-arrangements.pdf.

Koh, Katherine A, and Ann Elizabeth Montgomery. "Adverse Childhood Experiences and Homelessness: Advances and Aspirations." *The Lancet Public Health* 6, no. 11 (November 2021). https://doi.org/10.1016/s2468-2667(21)00210-3.

Koski, Jessica E., Hongling Xie, and Ingrid R. Olson. "Understanding Social Hierarchies: The Neural and Psychological Foundations of Status Perception." *Social Neuroscience* 10, no. 5 (February 20, 2015): 527–50. https://doi.org/10.1080/17470919.2015.1013223.

Kurani, Nisha, and Cynthia Cox. "What Drives Health Spending in the U.S. Compared to Other Countries." Peterson-KFF Health System Tracker, July 20, 2021. https://www.healthsystemtracker.org/brief/what-drives-health-spending-in-the-u-s-compared-to-other-countries/.

La Roche, Julia. "Buffett: 'Medical Costs Are the Tapeworm of American Economic Competitiveness.'" Yahoo! Finance. Accessed July 15, 2024. https://finance.yahoo.com/news/buffett-medical-costs-tapeworm-american-economic-competitiveness-220647855.html.

Larimer, Mary E., Bonnie Burlingham, David C Atkins, Michelle D Garner, Daniel K Malone, Joshua Ginzler, Kenneth Tanzer, et al. "Health Care and Public Service Use and Costs Before and After Provision of Housing for Chronically Homeless Persons with Severe Alcohol Problems." *JAMA* 301, no. 13 (April 1, 2009): 1349. https://doi.org/10.1001/jama.2009.414.

Levey, Noam N. "Few Places Have More Medical Debt than Dallas-Fort Worth, but Hospitals There Are Thriving." *KFF Health News*, September 30, 2022. https://khn.org/news/article/medical-debt-hospitals-dallas-fort-worth/.

Lichtenstein, Bronwen, and Joe Weber. "Losing Ground: Racial Disparities in Medical Debt and Home Foreclosure in the Deep South. Fam Community Health." *Family & Community Health* 39, no. 3 (July 2016): 178–87. https://doi.org/10.1097/fch.0000000000000108.

Linardon, Jake, Mariel Messer, Simon B. Goldberg, and Matthew Fuller-Tyszkiewicz. "The Efficacy of Mindfulness Apps on Symptoms of Depression and Anxiety: An Updated Meta-Analysis of Randomized Controlled Trials." *Clinical Psychology Review* 107 (February 2024): 102370. https://doi.org/10.1016/j.cpr.2023.102370.

Lockwood, Patricia L. "The Anatomy of Empathy: Vicarious Experience and Disorders of Social Cognition." *Behavioural Brain Research* 311 (September 2016): 255–66. https://doi.org/10.1016/j.bbr.2016.05.048.

Loomans, M M, J H M Tulen, and H J C van Marle. "The Neurobiology of Antisocial Behaviour." *Tijdschr Psychiatr*, 2010.

Lopez, Eric, Tricia Neuman, Gretchen Jacobson, and Larry Levitt. "How Much More Than Medicare Do Private Insurers Pay? A Review of the Literature." *KFF*, April 15, 2020.

Lount, Robert B., and Nathan C. Pettit. "The Social Context of Trust: The Role of Status." *Organizational Behavior and Human Decision Processes* 117, no. 1 (January 2012): 15–23. https://doi.org/10.1016/j.obhdp.2011.07.005.

Makary, Martin A, and Michael Daniel. "Medical Error—the Third Leading Cause of Death in the US." *BMJ*, May 3, 2016, i2139. https://doi.org/10.1136/bmj.i2139.

McGuire, Thomas G., and Jeanne Miranda. "New Evidence Regarding Racial and Ethnic Disparities in Mental Health: Policy Implications." *Health Affairs* 27, no. 2 (March 2008): 393–403. https://doi.org/10.1377/hlthaff.27.2.393.

"Medicare Access and Chip Reauthorization Act (Macra), H.R. 2." *Primary Care Collaborative*, April 1, 2015. https://www.pcpcc.org/resource/medicare-access-and-chip-reauthorization-act-macra-hr-2.

Melek, Stephen P, Sheri Kirshenbaum, Brian Klausner, and Von Nguyen. "Whole-

Person Health Care: Integrating Mental and Behavioral Health Into Primary Care." *The American Journal of Managed Care*. Lecture, October 16, 2020.

Morris, Zoë Slote, Steven Wooding, and Jonathan Grant. "The Answer Is 17 Years, What Is the Question: Understanding Time Lags in Translational Research." *Journal of the Royal Society of Medicine* 104, no. 12 (December 2011): 510–20. https://doi.org/10.1258/jrsm.2011.110180.

Naito, Ryo, Martin McKee, Darryl Leong, Shrikant Bangdiwala, Sumathy Rangarajan, Shofiqul Islam, and Salim Yusuf. "Social Isolation as a Risk Factor for All-Cause Mortality: Systematic Review and Meta-Analysis of Cohort Studies." *PLOS ONE* 18, no. 1 (January 12, 2023). https://doi.org/10.1371/journal.pone.0280308.

"New Maps Show Differences in Life Expectancy." *North Carolina Health News*, August 5, 2015. https://www.northcarolinahealthnews.org/2015/08/05/new-maps-show-differences-in-life-expectancy.

"NHE Fact Sheet." CMS.gov. Accessed July 15, 2024. https://www.cms.gov/data-research/statistics-trends-and-reports/national-health-expenditure-data/nhe-fact-sheet.

"North Carolina: All Race & Ethnicity Data." The COVID Tracking Project. Accessed July 15, 2024. https://covidtracking.com/data/state/north-carolina/race-ethnicity.

Office of Policy, Planning, and Innovation, SAMHSA's Concept of Trauma and Guidance for a Trauma-Informed Approach (2014).

Office of the Assistant Secretary for Health (OASH). "New Surgeon General Advisory Raises Alarm about the Devastating Impact of the Epidemic of Loneliness and Isolation in the United States." HHS.gov, May 3, 2023. https://www.hhs.gov/about/news/2023/05/03/new-surgeon-general-advisory-raises-alarm-about-devastating-impact-epidemic-loneliness-isolation-united-states.html.

Office of the Under Secretary of Defense, National Defense Budget Estimates for FY 2020 (2019).

Olson, LeighAnne, Robert S Sanders, and Pierre L Long. "The Healthcare Imperative: Lowering Costs and Improving Outcomes." *Institute of Medicine (US) Roundtable on Evidence-Based Medicine*, December 17, 2010. https://doi.org/10.17226/12750.

Oppong, Thomas. "Aristotle's Principles for a Good Life." *Medium*, September 21, 2022. https://medium.com/personal-growth/aristotles-principles-for-a-good-life-9f474a5f02bc.

O'Connell, James J. "Premature Mortality in Homeless Populations: A Review of the Literature." *National Health Care for the Homeless Council*, 2005.

Pear, Robert. "Clinton's Health Plan: The Overview; Congress Is given the Clinton Plan for Health Care." *The New York Times*, October 28, 1993.

Piff, Paul K., Daniel M. Stancato, Stéphane Côté, Rodolfo Mendoza-Denton, and Dacher Keltner. "Higher Social Class Predicts Increased Unethical Behavior." *Proceedings of the National Academy of Sciences* 109, no. 11 (February 27, 2012): 4086–91. https://doi.org/10.1073/pnas.1118373109.

Point in Time Data - 2021 - Wake Continuum of Care - NC 507. Accessed July 16, 2024. https://wakecoc.org/data/pit-2021/.

Portelli Tremont, Jaclyn N., Brian Klausner, and Pascal Osita Udekwu. "Embracing a Trauma-Informed Approach to Patient Care—in with the New." *JAMA Surgery* 156, no. 12 (December 1, 2021): 1083. https://doi.org/10.1001/jamasurg.2021.4284.

Published: May 01, 2012. "Health Care Costs: A Primer 2012 Report." KFF, July 25, 2014. https://www.kff.org/report-section/health-care-costs-a-primer-2012-report/.

Ramirez, Franchesca, Justin M. Moscarello, Joseph E. LeDoux, and Robert M. Sears. "Active Avoidance Requires a Serial Basal Amygdala to Nucleus Accumbens Shell Circuit." *The Journal of Neuroscience* 35, no. 8 (February 25, 2015): 3470–77. https://doi.org/10.1523/jneurosci.1331-14.2015.

Rep. *The Silent Shortage: A White Paper Examining Supply, Demand and Recruitment Trends in Psychiatry*. White Paper Series. Merritt Hawkins, 2018.

Rep. *Wake County Population Health Task Force*. Wake County, NC, 2018.

Rountree, Janey, Austen Lyke, and Nathan Hess. "Health Conditions among Unsheltered Adults in the U.S." California Policy Lab, October 6, 2019. https://capolicylab.org/health-conditions-among-unsheltered-adults-in-the-u-s/.

Schroeder, Steven A. "We Can Do Better—Improving the Health of the American People." *New England Journal of Medicine* 357, no. 12 (September 20, 2007): 1221–28. https://doi.org/10.1056/nejmsa073350.

Schwartz, Katrina. "Four Pillars of a Meaningful Life That Could Be Part of Every Learning Community." KQED, December 10, 2018. https://www.kqed.org/mindshift/52620/four-pillars-of-a-meaningful-life-that-could-be-part-of-every-learning-community.

Shrank, William H., Teresa L. Rogstad, and Natasha Parekh. "Waste in the US Health Care System." *JAMA* 322, no. 15 (October 15, 2019): 1501. https://doi.org/10.1001/jama.2019.13978.

Singh Ospina, Naykky, Kari A. Phillips, Rene Rodriguez-Gutierrez, Ana Castaneda-Guarderas, Michael R. Gionfriddo, Megan E. Branda, and Victor M. Montori. "Eliciting the Patient's Agenda- Secondary Analysis of Recorded Clinical Encounters." *Journal of General Internal Medicine* 34, no. 1 (July 2, 2018): 36–40. https://doi.org/10.1007/s11606-018-4540-5.

St Clair, William. *The Grand Slave Emporium: Cape Coast Castle and the British Slave Trade*. London: Profile Books, 2006.

"State of Homelessness: 2023 Edition." National Alliance to End Homelessness, January 6, 2024. https://endhomelessness.org/homelessness-in-america/homelessness-statistics/state-of-homelessness.

"Story Map Series." unc.maps.arcgis.com. Accessed July 15, 2024. https://unc.maps.arcgis.com/apps/MapSeries/index.html?appid=5eb9f9d962914ab19e5b454b30637104.

Thomsen, Lotte. "The Developmental Origins of Social Hierarchy: How Infants and Young Children Mentally Represent and Respond to Power and Status." *Current Opinion in Psychology* 33 (June 2020): 201–8. https://doi.org/10.1016/j.copsyc.2019.07.044.

Torres, Francis. "U.S. Opinions on Homelessness: A BPC/Morning Consult Poll."

Bipartisan Policy Center. June 5, 2023. https://bipartisanpolicy.org/blog/us-opinions-homelessness-poll.

Touroutoglou, Alexandra, Joseph Andreano, Bradford C. Dickerson, and Lisa Feldman Barrett. "The Tenacious Brain: How the Anterior Mid-Cingulate Contributes to Achieving Goals." *Cortex* 123 (February 2020): 12–29. https://doi.org/10.1016/j.cortex.2019.09.011.

US Department of Justice, and Caroline Wolf Harlow, Education and Correctional Populations (2003).

Udoetuk, Sade, Deepa Dongarwar, and Hamisu M. Salihu. "Racial and Gender Disparities in Diagnosis of Malingering in Clinical Settings." *Journal of Racial and Ethnic Health Disparities* 7, no. 6 (March 9, 2020): 1117–23. https://doi.org/10.1007/s40615-020-00734-6.

"Understanding the Impact of Adverse Childhood Experiences (ACEs)." Center for Youth Wellness, June 26, 2024. https://centerforyouthwellness.org/wp-content/themes/cyw/build/img/building-a-movement/hidden-crisis.pdf.

United States Interagency Council on Homelessness. "Homeless Courts: Recognizing Progress and Resolving Legal Issues That Often Accompany Homelessness." United States Interagency Council on Homelessness, July 9, 2020. https://www.usich.gov/news/homeless-courts-recognizing-progress-and-resolving-legal-issues-that-often-accompany-homelessness.

Vankar, Preeti. "US Health Expenditure as Percent of GDP from 1960 to 2022." Statista. February 16, 2024. https://www.statista.com/statistics/184968/us-health-expenditure-as-percent-of-gdp-since-1960

Waldinger, Robert. "What Makes a Good Life? Lessons from the Longest Study on Happiness." *TedxBeaconStreet*. Lecture, n.d. https://www.ted.com/talks/robert_waldinger_what_makes_a_good_life_lessons_from_the_longest_study_on_happiness.

Weiner, Jonathan P., Stephen Bandeian, Elham Hatef, Daniel Lans, Angela Liu, and Klaus W. Lemke. "In-Person and Telehealth Ambulatory Contacts and Costs in a Large US Insured Cohort before and during the COVID-19 Pandemic." *JAMA Network Open* 4, no. 3 (March 23, 2021). https://doi.org/10.1001/jamanetworkopen.2021.2618.

Wenzel, Suzanne L., Barbara D. Leake, and Lillian Gelberg. "Health of Homeless Women with Recent Experience of Rape." *Journal of General Internal Medicine* 15, no. 4 (April 2000): 265–68. https://doi.org/10.1111/j.1525-1497.2000.04269.x.

"What Are Adverse Childhood Experiences (Aces)?" WAVE Trust. Accessed July 15, 2024. https://www.wavetrust.org/adverse-childhood-experiences.

Working paper. *Early Experiences Can Alter Gene Expression and Affect Long-Term Development*, 2010.

Young, Amy M., Carol Boyd, and Amy Hubbell. "Social Isolation & Sexual Abuse among Women Who Smoke Crack." *Journal of Psychosocial Nursing and Mental Health Services* 39, no. 7 (July 2001): 12–20. https://doi.org/10.3928/0279-3695-20010701-10.

THANK YOU!

I wanted to publish *In the Gaps* by 2022. It did not quite work out, as I slightly underestimated how challenging it was to actually write a book. Over the years that it took me to finish *In the Gaps*, homelessness across our nation, and specifically in my city of Raleigh, got worse. Much worse. Numbers are now at a record high.

I've also learned that once a book is complete, the process of going through a traditional publisher can add years to the process and carries a risk of losing autonomy over final content.

I didn't want to lose any more time. I definitely did not want to lose autonomy. So I decided to publish independently, which honestly has been awesome and really fun.

Without a publisher's support, however, I will be dependent on social media, word of mouth, and reviews to spread the word. If you enjoyed the book, you will have my sincere gratitude if you can leave a review on Amazon. If you did not enjoy the book, you will have my sincere apologies (I tried!). Either way, thank you for reading!

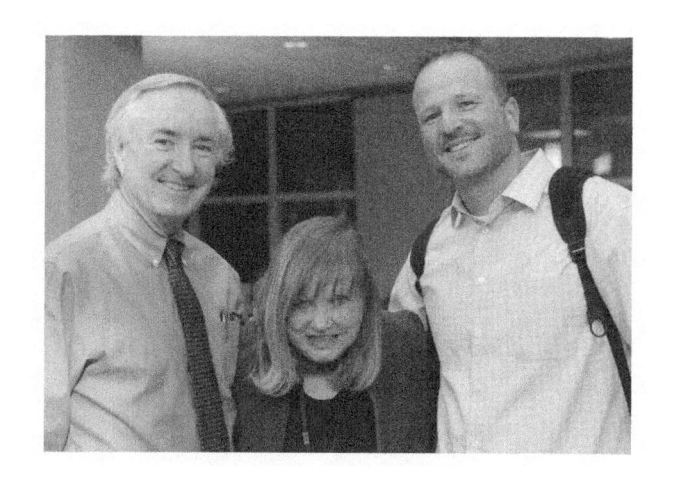

Jim O'Connell, Joanne Guarino, and Brian Klausner in 2017 at Boston Health Care for the Homeless

ABOUT THE AUTHOR

Dr. Brian Klausner has spent his career advocating for patients and driving quality improvement, with a specific interest in high-risk populations.

Born and raised in Los Angeles, Dr. Brian Klausner graduated from the University of Notre Dame and then Georgetown University School of Medicine, where he attended as a National Health Service Corp Scholar. Following the completion of his internal medicine training at the University of Chicago, he joined the Boston Health Care for the Homeless Program, eventually becoming the medical director of its largest outpatient clinic.

After moving to Raleigh in 2011, Dr. Klausner continued in his population-health leadership roles at WakeMed Hospital, eventually serving as the chief medical officer of WakeMed Key Community Care Accountable Care Organization. Simultaneously during that time, Dr. Klausner developed and led North Carolina's first "hotspotter" model designed to identify and better manage Wake County's highest-risk, highest-cost uninsured patients. In the context of his experience with evolving trauma-informed models, Dr. Klausner has also served as a partner physician for HostageUS since 2020.

In October 2022, Dr. Klausner helped to establish WakeMed's Center for Community Health, Innovation, and Equity, where clinical teams manage high-risk patients while also developing innovative community collaborations designed to address local health inequities.

Dr. Klausner and his clinical models have won numerous awards throughout his career and have been featured in numerous medical and news outlets including *Politico*, *USA Today*, NPR, and *Modern Healthcare*, as have various editorials he has written over the years.